Clinical Pharmacology and Therapeutics:
Questions for Self Assessment

THIRD EDITION

TIMOTHY GK MANT BSc FFPM FRCP
Senior Medical Advisor, Quintiles, Guy's Drug Research Unit, and
Visiting Professor, King's College London School of Medicine at Guys,
King's and St Thomas' Hospitals, London, UK

LIONEL D LEWIS MA MB BCh MD FRCP
Professor of Medicine, Pharmacology and Toxicology at Dartmouth
Medical School and the Dartmouth-Hitchcock Medical Center,
Lebanon, New Hampshire, USA

JAMES M RITTER MA DPhil FRCP FMedSci FBPHARMACOLS
Professor of Clinical Pharmacology, King's College London School of
Medicine at Guy's, King's and St Thomas' Hospitals, London, UK

ALBERT FERRO PhD FRCP FBPHARMACOLS
Reader in Clinical Pharmacology and Honorary Consultant
Physician, King's College London School of Medicine at Guy's,
King's and St Thomas' Hospitals, London, UK

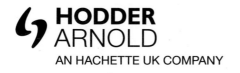

**HODDER
ARNOLD**
AN HACHETTE UK COMPANY

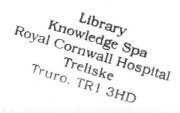

First published in Great Britain in 1995 as *Multiple Choice Questions in Clinical Pharmacology*
Second edition published in 2000
This third edition published in Great Britain in 2008 by
Hodder Arnold, an imprint of Hodder Education,
an Hachette UK Company, 338 Euston Road, London NW1 3BH

http://www.hoddereducation.com

Hodder Education's policy is to use papers that are natural, renewable and recyclable products
and made from wood grown in sustainable forests. The logging and manufacturing processes are
expected to conform to the environmental regulations of the country of origin.

Whilst the advice and information in this book are believed to be true and accurate at the date of
going to press, neither the authors nor the publisher can accept any legal responsibility or liability
for any errors or omissions that may be made. In particular, (but without limiting the generality of
the preceding disclaimer) every effort has been made to check drug dosages; however it is still
possible that errors have been missed. Furthermore, dosage schedules are constantly being
revised and new side-effects recognized. For these reasons the reader is strongly urged to consult
the drug companies' printed instructions before administering any of the drugs recommended in
this book.

British Library Cataloguing in Publication Data
A catalogue record for this book is available from the British Library

Library of Congress Cataloging-in-Publication Data
A catalog record for this book is available from the Library of Congress

ISBN   978–0–340–94743–2

3 4 5 6 7 8 9 10

Commissioning Editor: Sara Purdy
Project Editor: Jane Tod
Production Controller: Andre Sim
Cover Design: Laura de Grasse

Typeset in 9/11.5 Palatino by Charon Tec Ltd (A Macmillan Company),
Chennai, India
Printed and bound in India

What do you think about this book? Or any other Hodder Arnold title?
Please visit our website: www.hoddereducation.com

CONTENTS

INTRODUCTION   v

1 GENERAL PRINCIPLES   1

Multiple Choice Questions   1
Extended Matching Questions   15
Answers   19

2 NERVOUS SYSTEM   39

Multiple Choice Questions   39
Extended Matching Questions   53
Answers   55

3 MUSCULOSKELETAL SYSTEM   69

Multiple Choice Questions   69
Extended Matching Questions   71
Answers   72

4 CARDIOVASCULAR SYSTEM   75

Multiple Choice Questions   75
Extended Matching Questions   86
Answers   89

5 RESPIRATORY SYSTEM   101

Multiple Choice Questions   101
Extended Matching Questions   104
Answers   105

6 ALIMENTARY SYSTEM   109

Multiple Choice Questions   109
Extended Matching Questions   115
Answers   116

7 ENDOCRINE SYSTEM   122

Multiple Choice Questions   122
Extended Matching Questions   127
Answers   129

8 SELECTIVE TOXICITY   135

Multiple Choice Questions   135
Extended Matching Questions   144
Answers   147

9 CLINICAL IMMUNOPHARMACOLOGY   159

Multiple Choice Questions   159
Extended Matching Questions   162
Answers   163

10 THE SKIN AND THE EYE   167

Multiple Choice Questions   167
Extended Matching Questions   170
Answers   171

11 CLINICAL TOXICOLOGY   174

Multiple Choice Questions   174
Extended Matching Questions   178
Answers   179

12 PRACTICE EXAMINATION   184

Best of Fives   184
Problem solving questions   197
Answers   202

INTRODUCTION

Multiple choice, extended matching, best of five and problem solving questions are now ubiquitous in medical graduate and postgraduate examinations. They provide a rapid method for testing a wide range of knowledge and marking is objective. The authors of this book, who are all practising physicians who have taught clinical pharmacology and therapeutics for many years, have based it on the fifth edition of *Textbook of Clinical Pharmacology and Therapeutics* not only to prepare students for their exams but also to emphasize the principles and facts that are the key to safe and effective prescribing.

The answers are related to the relevant section in *Textbook of Clinical Pharmacology and Therapeutics*, Fifth Edition. In addition there are brief explanatory annotations in the answer to each question.

Although this book can 'stand alone', we recommend that students will read a section of the main textbook and then reinforce and revise their knowledge by self testing using the self assessment book. At the end of the book is a practice examination of 50 'Best one correct answer of five' questions, the type currently most favoured in medical examinations, followed by five problem solving questions. This examination covers the spectrum of topics that may be encountered in a final MB (medical degree) examination or even in some postgraduate examinations (e.g. American Board of Clinical Pharmacology, Inc.). We suggest that students use this as a 'practice run' after finishing their revision of the subject as a whole. It is best to do it 'blind' at one sitting lasting not more than 60 minutes.

We thank the generations of students who have provided critical feedback and Val Brockwell for her word processing skills and patience.

Timothy Mant
Lionel Lewis
James Ritter
Albert Ferro

CHAPTER ONE

GENERAL PRINCIPLES

MULTIPLE CHOICE QUESTIONS

1 The following drugs exert their effects by binding to receptors and mimicking the effects of the endogenous ligand (i.e. are agonists):

a) Tamoxifen
b) Salbutamol
c) Morphine
d) Cetirizine
e) Lisinopril

2 The following drugs exert their principal effects by enzyme inhibition:

a) Pyridostigmine
b) Atropine
c) Amlodipine
d) Digoxin
e) Selegiline

3 The following drugs are reversible competitive antagonists:

a) Suxamethonium
b) Loratidine
c) Ranitidine
d) Phenoxybenzamine
e) Naloxone

4 The following drugs are partial agonists:

a) Isoprenaline
b) Morphine
c) Flumazenil
d) Buprenorphine
e) Oxprenolol

5　The following drugs cause their primary pharmacodynamic effect via non-receptor mediated mechanisms:

a) Magnesium trisilicate
b) Mannitol
c) Methotrexate
d) Dimercaprol
e) Sumatriptan

6　The pharmacokinetic 'elimination half-life' of the following drugs mirrors their pharmacodynamic duration and intensity of action:

a) Salbutamol
b) Phenelzine
c) Dobutamine
d) Omeprazole
e) Cyclophosphamide

7　The plasma clearance of a drug:

a) Is the volume of plasma from which the drug is totally eliminated per unit time
b) Is equal to the administration rate divided by the steady state plasma concentration
c) Is a better measure of the efficiency of drug elimination from the body than elimination half-life
d) Does not include elimination by hepatic enzyme metabolism
e) May be affected by renal function (i.e. GFR)

8　For a drug that obeys first-order (linear) kinetics and fits a one-compartment model for elimination:

a) Its rate of elimination (in mass units of drug/unit time) is proportional to its plasma concentration
b) Following cessation of an intravenous infusion the plasma concentration declines exponentially
c) The half-life is proportional to the dose
d) The half-life is unaffected by renal function (i.e. GFR)
e) The composition of drug products excreted is independent of the dose

9　The apparent volume of distribution:

a) Can be greater than the total body volume
b) Is approximately 3 L for most drugs in adults
c) Is influenced by a drug's lipid solubility
d) A large value indicates that a drug will be efficiently eliminated by haemodialysis
e) Determines the peak plasma concentration after a single bolus intravenous dose

10 The following drugs have an elimination half-life of less than 4 hours in a healthy adult:

   a) Dopamine
   b) Heparin
   c) Amiodarone
   d) Gentamicin
   e) Diazepam

11 In repeated (chronic or multiple) dosing:

   a) If the dosing interval is much greater than the elimination half-life, little if any drug accumulation occurs
   b) It takes approximately five half-lives to reach 50 per cent of the steady state concentration
   c) If a drug is administered once every half-life once steady state is reached, the peak plasma concentration will be double the trough concentration
   d) The use of a bolus loading dose reduces the time taken to reach steady state
   e) In patients with renal impairment the dosing interval should be increased when prescribing gentamicin

12 The following drugs obey non-linear (dose-dependent) elimination pharmacokinetics:

   a) Acetylsalicylic acid (aspirin) overdose
   b) Heparin
   c) Phenytoin
   d) Ethanol
   e) Ceftazidime in therapeutic doses

13 The following drugs undergo significant enterohepatic circulation:

   a) Oestrogens
   b) Atenolol
   c) Rifampicin
   d) Gentamicin
   e) Levofloxacin

14 The oral bioavailability of a drug:

   a) Is a measure of the extent to which it enters the systemic circulation
   b) May be influenced by changing the excipient after oral administration
   c) Is defined as the ratio of the area under the plasma concentration time curve (AUC) following oral administration divided by that following intravenous administration
   d) May be reduced by hepatic CYP450 induction
   e) Two preparations of the same drug may have similar bioavailability but different peak concentrations (C_{max})

15 The following are examples of prodrugs:
- a) Levodopa
- b) Azathioprine
- c) Penciclovir
- d) Sulfasalazine
- e) Enalapril

16 The following oral drugs do not require absorption from the gut to exert a therapeutic effect:
- a) Acarbose
- b) Methionine
- c) Orlistat
- d) Olsalazine
- e) Vancomycin

17 Drug absorption following oral administration:
- a) Is most commonly through passive diffusion
- b) Occurs predominantly in the colon
- c) Is usually complete within 90 minutes
- d) Non-polar lipid-soluble drugs are absorbed more readily than polar water-soluble drugs
- e) Peptides are well absorbed following oral administration

18 The following drugs are absorbed predominantly through active transport systems:
- a) Paracetamol (acetaminophen)
- b) Phenytoin
- c) Levodopa
- d) Methyldopa
- e) Lithium

19 The systemic bioavailability of the following oral drugs is increased if taken in the fasting state:
- a) Oxytetracycline
- b) Amoxicillin
- c) Levodopa
- d) Acetylsalicylic acid/salicylates
- e) Fluconazole

20 The following drugs are effectively administered via the sublingual route:
- a) Simvastatin
- b) Carbamazepine
- c) Ramipril
- d) Buprenorphine
- e) Glyceryl trinitrate

21   The following drugs are effectively administered by the rectal route to produce their systemic effect:

a) Indometacin
b) Sulfasalazine
c) Metronidazole
d) Glycerin
e) Diazepam

22   The following drugs may be administered transcutaneously to produce their systemic therapeutic effect:

a) Glyceryl trinitrate (GTN)
b) Estradiol
c) Lidocaine (lignocaine)
d) Fentanyl
e) Nicotine

23   In the case of an intramuscular injection of a drug:

a) Rate of drug absorption is enhanced by exercise
b) Rate of drug absorption is greater from the deltoid injection site than the gluteus maximus site
c) If administered to the buttock should be in the upper outer quadrant
d) Should usually be no greater than a volume of 0.5 mL
e) Is an appropriate route of administration for the decanoate ester of fluphenazine

24   The following are commonly associated with phlebitis when given via the intravenous route:

a) Potassium chloride
b) Hydrocortisone
c) Diazepam
d) 50 per cent glucose
e) 5 per cent glucose

25   The following are metabolized by enzymes in the hepatic smooth endoplasmic reticulum:

a) Levodopa
b) Tyramine
c) Metoprolol
d) Suxamethonium
e) 6-Mercaptopurine

26   The following are substrates for CYP3A:

a) Ciclosporin
b) Clarithromycin
c) Phenytoin
d) Adrenaline (epinephrine)
e) Warfarin

27 The following drugs undergo phase II metabolism by hepatic acetylation enzymes (N-acetyltransferases):

a) Dapsone
b) Ciclosporin
c) Gentamicin
d) Isoniazid
e) Hydralazine

28 The following agents induce hepatic CYP450:

a) Rifampicin
b) Carbamazepine
c) St John's wort
d) Phenobarbital
e) Penicillin

29 The following inhibit at least one of the hepatic CYP450 isoenzymes:

a) Fluvoxamine
b) Grapefruit juice
c) Digoxin
d) Itraconazole
e) Ciprofloxacin

30 The following are subject to extensive presystemic (first-pass) metabolism:

a) Metoprolol
b) Phenytoin
c) Ciprofloxacin
d) Morphine
e) Verapamil

31 The following decrease the rate of gastric emptying:

a) Aspirin overdose
b) Migraine
c) Fluoxetine
d) Amitriptyline
e) Metoclopramide

32 Cardiac failure:

a) Increases the bioavailability of oral thiazide diuretics
b) Increases the volume of distribution of lidocaine
c) Has little effect on the volume of distribution of furosemide
d) Decreases the elimination half-life of lidocaine
e) Decreases the elimination half-life of gentamicin

33 In severe renal failure:

a) Gastric pH decreases
b) The 'therapeutic range' for phenytoin decreases
c) Drug distribution of famotidine to the brain is increased
d) Smaller maintenance doses of digoxin are required
e) Omeprazole should be avoided

34 The following statements concerning renal drug handling are correct:

a) The kidneys receive approximately 20 per cent of the cardiac output
b) In healthy young adults approximately 130 mL/min of protein-free filtrate is formed at the glomeruli
c) Non-protein-bound drug of molecular weight <66 000 passes into the filtrate
d) Potentially saturable mechanisms for active secretion of both acids and bases exist in the proximal tubule
e) Low lipid solubility favours tubular reabsorption

35 The following drugs must be avoided in severe renal failure (glomerular filtration rate (GFR) <10 mL/min):

a) Prednisolone
b) Amoxicillin
c) Bumetanide
d) Metformin
e) Oxytetracycline

36 The following can reduce GFR:

a) Naproxen
b) Ranitidine
c) Iodine-containing contrast media
d) Lisinopril
e) Amphotericin B

37 Monitoring plasma/serum drug concentrations of the following drugs is recognized as a valuable supplement to clinical monitoring:

a) Carbimazole
b) Warfarin
c) Gentamicin
d) Lithium
e) Ciclosporin

38 In pregnancy:

a) Most drugs cross the placenta by active transport
b) Ionized drugs cross the placenta more easily than un-ionized drugs
c) Drugs that reduce placental blood flow can reduce birth weight
d) The fetal blood–brain barrier is not developed until the second half of pregnancy
e) The human placenta metabolizes endogenous steroids

39 The following drugs are confirmed teratogens in humans:
   a) Ethanol (alcohol)
   b) Warfarin
   c) Isotretinoin
   d) Paracetamol (acetaminophen)
   e) Amoxicillin

40 During pregnancy:
   a) Gastric emptying and small intestinal motility are reduced
   b) Blood volume increases
   c) Plasma volume increases
   d) Predominantly water-soluble drugs will have a larger apparent volume of distribution
   e) Phenytoin metabolism is inhibited

41 During pregnancy:
   a) Renal plasma flow increases
   b) GFR increases
   c) Atenolol excretion increases
   d) Lithium excretion increases
   e) Gentamicin excretion increases

42 The following are considered safe during pregnancy:
   a) Salbutamol
   b) Erythromycin
   c) Levofloxacin
   d) Tobramycin
   e) Ribavirin

43 The following are appropriate in the management of benign dyspepsia in the second and third trimester of pregnancy:
   a) Low roughage diet
   b) Avoidance of fresh fruit and vegetables
   c) Small, frequent meals
   d) Misoprostol
   e) Omeprazole

44 The following drugs do not cross the placenta in significant amounts:
   a) Heparin
   b) Warfarin
   c) Corticosteroids
   d) Sodium valproate
   e) Pethidine

45 The use of phenytoin in pregnancy:
   a) Is absolutely contraindicated
   b) Is associated with cleft lip and palate
   c) The 'therapeutic' blood concentration of total drug is lower than in the non-pregnant state
   d) Is associated with ataxia if an excessive dose is used
   e) Requires oral vitamin D supplements

46 The following drugs are appropriate for managing severe hypertension diagnosed in early pregnancy in an asthmatic woman:
   a) Bendromethiazide
   b) Atenolol
   c) Labetalol
   d) Lisinopril
   e) Methyldopa

47 The following are absolutely contraindicated in pregnancy:
   a) Salbutamol
   b) Corticosteroids
   c) General anaesthesia
   d) Quinine for malaria
   e) Sucralfate

48 In neonates relative to adults:
   a) Gastric acid production is reduced
   b) Fat content (as a percentage of body weight) is low
   c) Plasma albumin concentration is low
   d) The blood–brain barrier is more permeable
   e) The GFR is reduced

49 The following drugs should be avoided during breastfeeding:
   a) Amiodarone
   b) Carbamazepine
   c) Ciprofloxacin
   d) Cyclophosphamide
   e) Ranitidine

50 The following drugs suppress lactation:
   a) Anthraquinones (e.g. senna)
   b) Bromocriptine
   c) Furosemide
   d) Salbutamol
   e) Metronidazole

51 The following properties of a drug facilitate its entry into breast milk:

a) High lipid solubility
b) Un-ionized state at physiological pH
c) Low molecular weight
d) Weak base
e) Short half-life

52 The following are appropriate in the first-line management of acute severe asthma in a 5-year-old child:

a) Nebulized beta$_2$ agonists
b) Systemic corticosteroids
c) Rectal diazepam
d) Systemic ipratropium
e) Systemic midazolam

53 A 'normal' man of 75 in comparison with a 'normal' man of 35:

a) Is more likely to be on regular drug therapy
b) Is more prone to sedation with benzodiazepines
c) Has a higher endogenous production of creatinine
d) Has an increased liability to allergic drug reactions
e) Usually requires a lower dose of warfarin to achieve anticoagulation

54 The following drugs may precipitate acute retention of urine in the elderly:

a) Gliclazide
b) Furosemide
c) Morphine
d) Amitriptyline
e) Trimethoprim

55 The half-life of the following is increased in the elderly:

a) Gentamicin
b) Glibenclamide
c) Lithium
d) Morphine glucuronide
e) Diazepam

56 The following drugs should not be used in patients over 75 years old:

a) Trandolapril
b) Finasteride
c) Streptokinase
d) Doxycycline
e) Fluoxetine

57 A woman of 75 is more likely to have the following adverse effects than a woman of 25:
- **a)** Confusion during treatment with cimetidine
- **b)** Cholestatic jaundice following treatment with flucloxacillin
- **c)** Gastrointestinal haemorrhage during treatment with ketorolac
- **d)** Increased incidence of postural hypotension during doxazosin therapy
- **e)** Increased risk of agranulocytosis during clozapine therapy

58 The following are 'type A' adverse reactions (i.e. a consequence of the drug's normal pharmacological effect):
- **a)** Propranolol and fatigue
- **b)** Atorvastatin and hepatotoxicity
- **c)** Naproxen and gastrointestinal haemorrhage
- **d)** Cyclophosphamide and neutropenia
- **e)** Diazepam and sedation

59 Stopping treatment with the following drugs may lead to adverse effects due to drug withdrawal:
- **a)** Prednisolone
- **b)** Clonidine
- **c)** Lorazepam
- **d)** Metoprolol
- **e)** Ergotamine

60 The following adverse reactions are associated with the drugs named:
- **a)** Oral contraception – gastrointestinal haemorrhage
- **b)** Co-amoxiclav – acute liver failure
- **c)** Cocaine – stroke
- **d)** Thiazide diuretics – impotence
- **e)** Prednisolone – osteomalacia

61 The following are examples of a type I hypersensitivity reaction:
- **a)** Penicillin-induced anaphylactic shock
- **b)** Methyldopa-induced Coombs' positive haemolytic anaemia
- **c)** Hydralazine-induced systemic lupus erythematosus (SLE)
- **d)** Amiodarone-induced photosensitivity skin rashes
- **e)** Sotalol-induced torsade de pointes

62 The following drugs are associated with erythema multiforme:
- **a)** Phenytoin
- **b)** Cyclophosphamide
- **c)** Salbutamol
- **d)** Sevoflurane
- **e)** Co-trimoxazole

63 The following drugs are recognized as causing thrombocytopenia:
a) Aurothiomalate
b) Thiazides
c) Heparin
d) Mesalazine
e) Atenolol

64 The following combinations outside the body (e.g. in infusion bag) cause drug inactivation:
a) Penicillin and hydrocortisone
b) Phenytoin and 5 per cent dextrose
c) Sodium bicarbonate and calcium chloride
d) Erythromycin and 0.9 per cent sodium chloride
e) Heparin and 5 per cent dextrose

65 Individuals who are 'slow acetylators' (i.e. have relatively low activities of hepatic N-acetyltransferase):
a) Have prevalence of 5–10 per cent amongst the white population in the UK
b) Are more likely to develop agranulocytosis whilst being treated with clozapine
c) Are more likely to develop hepatotoxicity after a paracetamol overdose
d) Are more likely to develop a lupus-like syndrome during hydralazine therapy
e) Are more likely to develop peripheral neuropathy during isoniazid therapy

66 The following drugs can produce haemolysis in patients with glucose 6-phosphate dehydrogenase (G6PD) deficiency:
a) Dapsone
b) Probenecid
c) Primaquine
d) Co-trimoxazole
e) Ciprofloxacin

67 Drug-induced exacerbations of acute porphyria:
a) Are usually precipitated by enzyme inhibitors (e.g. selegiline)
b) Are often precipitated by a single dose of drug
c) Are accompanied by increased urinary excretion of 5-aminolevulinic acid (ALA) and porphobilinogen
d) May be precipitated by ethanol
e) May be precipitated by rifampicin

68 Abnormal pseudocholinesterase:

a) Is typically inherited as a Mendelian dominant condition

b) Results in malignant hyperthermia following exposure to suxamethonium

c) Causes warfarin resistance

d) Leads to prolonged paralysis following suxamethonium

e) Is associated with treatment failure with donepezil for Alzheimer's disease

69 Phase 1 studies (i.e. initial studies of drugs in humans involving an Investigational Medicinal Product) in the UK:

a) Require authorization by the Medicines and Healthcare Products Regulatory Agency (MHRA)

b) The control group is usually the current drug of choice for the proposed indication

c) Always use the oral route of administration

d) Only commence after all animal studies have been completed

e) Are usually performed in patients who are asymptomatic with a terminal disease

70 The MHRA:

a) Is an independent group of clinicians, clinical pharmacologists, toxicologists, pathologists and others who advise the drug licensing authority

b) Is financed directly by the pharmaceutical industry

c) Considers the quality, safety and efficacy of medicinal products

d) Considers the investigation, monitoring and response to adverse reactions once a drug has been licensed

e) Appoints the committees on ethical practice, which assess drug trials

71 The following adverse reactions should be reported to the MHRA using the yellow card system:

a) A transient mild skin rash in a patient taking a new non-steroidal anti-inflammatory drug (NSAID) marked with a 'black triangle' in the *British National Formulary (BNF)*

b) Aggravation of asthma in a known asthmatic with the drug involved in question 'a' above

c) A convulsion following pertussis vaccination

d) Acute anaphylactic shock leading to death following intravenous benzylpenicillin

e) Fatal agranulocytosis associated with clozapine

72   The following licensed drugs are produced by insertion of human genes into bacterial, yeast or mammalian cell lines:

   a) Human insulin
   b) Growth hormone
   c) Factor VII
   d) Erythropoietin
   e) Interferon

Answers: see pages 19–33

EXTENDED MATCHING QUESTIONS

73 PHARMACODYNAMICS

A	Omeprazole	F	Atenolol
B	Clopidogrel	G	Dobutamine
C	Morphine	H	Warfarin
D	Glucagon	I	Magnesium trisilicate
E	Fluoxetine	J	Insulin

Select the drug that causes the pharmacodynamic effect described below:

1　Prolongation of prothrombin time
2　Reduction in blood glucose
3　Reduction in exercise-induced increase in heart rate
4　Pupil constriction
5　Inhibition of gastric acid secretion

74 PHARMACOKINETICS

A	Prednisolone	F	Metoprolol
B	Amiodarone	G	Simvastatin
C	Carbamazepine	H	Paracetamol
D	Lithium	I	Gentamicin
E	Enalapril	J	Bendroflumethiazide

Choose the drug from the list above which is a good example for the pharma-cokinetic characteristics listed below:

1　Absorption into the systemic circulation following oral administration is minimal
2　The mean elimination half-life is greater than 28 days in someone with normal hepatic and renal function
3　Is a prodrug which is hydrolysed to its active metabolite
4　Induces its own metabolism such that plasma concentrations may reduce significantly on repeated dosing
5　Undergoes active tubular reabsorption

75 PHARMACOGENETICS

A	Warfarin	F	Sildenafil
B	Digoxin	G	Suxamethonium
C	Omeprazole	H	Isoniazid
D	Cefuroxime	I	Heparin
E	Fluconazole	J	Codeine

Match the drug from the above list whose metabolism is most affected by the enzyme genetic polymorphism below:

1   CYP2D6
2   CYP2C9
3   N-Acetyltransferase
4   Pseudocholinesterase
5   CYP2CI9

76 ABSORPTION AND ROUTE OF ADMINISTRATION

A	Digoxin tablets	F	Levodopa
B	Intravenous insulin	G	Prednisolone
C	Glyceryl trinitrate	H	Methotrexate
D	Aspirin preparations	I	Diltiazem preparations
E	Simvastatin preparations	J	Rectal diazepam

Link each of 1 to 5 below with the most appropriate item from A to J:

1   Unsuitable for generic substitution
2   Bioavailability is 100 per cent
3   Prodrug
4   Sublingual administration circumvents extensive presystemic metabolism
5   Intrathecal injection is used in childhood leukaemia because of poor penetration of the blood–brain barrier

77 DRUG METABOLISM

A	Azathioprine	F	Rimonabant
B	Irinotecan	G	Midazolam
C	Clozapine	H	Amoxicillin
D	Dalteparin	I	Isoniazid
E	Phenylephrine	J	Warfarin

Choose the drug from the list above which is significantly affected by the enzyme below:

1   Monoamine oxidase
2   CYP1A2
3   CYP3A4
4   Uridine diphosphoglucuronyl transferase (UGT1AI)
5   Thiopurine methyltransferase (TPMT)

78 RENAL ELIMINATION

A	Clarithromycin	F	Lithium
B	Para-aminohippuric acid	G	Gentamicin
C	Probenecid	H	Senna
D	Salicylate	I	Thyroxine
E	Atorvastatin	J	Orlistat

Link each of 1 to 5 below with the most appropriate item from A to J:

1 Depends mainly on renal elimination
2 Competes for organic anion transport (OAT)
3 Excretion is enhanced by high urinary pH
4 Shares a proximal tubular transporter with Na^+
5 Is used to measure renal plasma flow

79 RENAL TRACT

A	Sildenafil	F	Acetazolamide
B	Finasteride	G	Bendroflumethiazide
C	Furosemide	H	Eplerenone
D	Oxybutinin	I	Desmopressin
E	Spironolactone	J	Tamsulosin

Link each of 1 to 5 below with the most appropriate drug from A to J:

1 Causes proximal renal tubular acidosis (RTA)
2 Oestrogen-related adverse effects
3 Blocks distal tubular Na^+/Cl^- reabsorption
4 Enhances ototoxicity of gentamicin
5 Adverse interaction with glyceryl trinitrate

80 ADVERSE DRUG REACTIONS

A	Gentamicin	F	Isoniazid
B	Amoxicillin	G	Spironolactone
C	Simvastatin	H	Clarithromycin
D	Prednisolone	I	Fluoxetine
E	Salbutamol	J	Flupentixol

For each adverse drug reaction match a likely causative drug:

1 Gynaecomastia
2 Osteoporosis
3 Myositis
4 SLE-like syndrome
5 Tardive dyskinesia

81 MONOCLONAL ANTIBODIES

A	Infliximab	**F**	Abciximab
B	Bevacizumab	**G**	Omalizumab
C	Basilixumab	**H**	Alemtuzumab
D	Anti-D (Rh) immunoglobulin	**I**	Rituximab
E	Natalizumab	**J**	Palivizumab

Match the monoclonal antibody with the mode of action described below:

1 Binds to respiratory syncytial virus
2 Anti IgE
3 Anti-tumour necrosis factor alpha (TNF-α)
4 Inhibition of vascular endothelial growth factor (VEGF)
5 Inhibition of glycoprotein IIb–IIIa

ANSWERS: see pages 33–38

MCQ ANSWERS

1 **a)** False – Tamoxifen is an anti-oestrogen which binds to the oestrogen receptor in breast tissue and inhibits oestrogen action and is used in breast cancer
   b) True – Salbutamol is a beta agonist. It is relatively selective for $beta_2$ effects (bronchodilation) but at higher doses $beta_1$ effects (tachycardia and tremor) also occur
   c) True – Morphine mimics the endogenous encephalins
   d) False – Cetirizine is an antihistamine (H_1 blocker)
   e) False – Lisinopril is an angiotensin-converting enzyme (ACE) inhibitor

2 **a)** True – Pyridostigmine is an inhibitor of acetylcholinesterase and is used in myasthenia gravis
   b) False – Atropine blocks muscarinic receptors
   c) False – Amlodipine is a calcium channel blocker
   d) True – Digoxin inhibits Na^+/K^+ adenosine triphosphatase (ATPase)
   e) True – Selegiline is a monoamine oxidase B (MAO-B) inhibitor used in Parkinson's disease

3 **a)** False – Suxamethonium is an agonist that causes a seemingly paradoxical inhibitory effect (neuromuscular blockade) by causing long-lasting depolarization of the neuromuscular junction
   b) True – Loratidine is a histamine (H_1) antagonist
   c) True – Ranitidine is a competitive histamine (H_2) antagonist
   d) False – Phenoxybenzamine is an irreversible alpha-receptor antagonist
   e) True – Naloxone is a competitive antagonist at the opiate mu-receptor

4 **a)** False Partial agonists combine with receptors but are incapable
   b) False of eliciting a maximal response whatever their
   c) False concentration (see *Textbook of Clinical Pharmacology and Therapeutics*, Chapter 2)
   d) True – Buprenorphine is a partial agonist at the opiate mu-receptor
   e) True – Oxprenolol is a partial agonist at the beta-adrenoceptor

5 **a)** True – Magnesium trisilicate is an antacid which neutralizes gastric acid

    b) True – Mannitol is an osmotic diuretic

    c) True – Methotrexate is a competitive inhibitor of dihydrofolate reductase and inhibits folate metabolism

    d) True – Dimercaprol is a chelating agent used in heavy metal poisoning

    e) False – Sumatriptan is a $5HT_{1D}$ agonist used in migraine

6 **a)** True   The magnitude of pharmacological effect usually depends

    b) False directly on the concentration of drug (or active metabolites)

    c) True   in the vicinity of their receptors. However, some drugs

    d) False bind to their target irreversibly so their effects

    e) False outlast their presence at these sites (e.g. alkylating agents at DNA)

7 **a)** True   Clearance and not half-life should be used as a measure of

    b) True   the efficiency of drug elimination

    c) True

    d) False

    e) True

8 **a)** True   Although the one-compartment model is an

    b) True   oversimplification, once absorption and distribution are

    c) False complete many drugs do obey first-order elimination

    d) False kinetics. See Fig. 1

    e) True

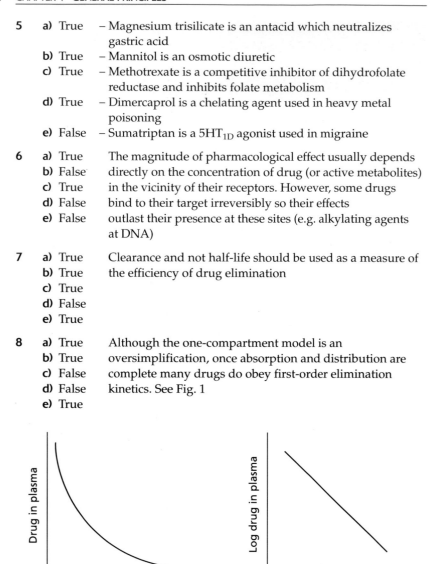

Fig. 1 One-compartment model. Plasma concentration-time curve following a bolus dose of drug plotted (a) arithmetically, or (b) semi-logarithmically. This drug fits a one-compartment model, i.e. its concentration falls exponentially with time.

9 **a)** True   Volume of distribution = dose/C_0, where C_0 is the plasma

    b) False concentration at time 0 calculated by extrapolation of the

    c) True   log concentration versus time relationship back to zero

 d) False   following a bolus intravenous injection. 3 L is the
 e) True   approximate total plasma volume in an adult

10 **a)** True   – Dopamine t½, 2 minutes
 b) True   – Heparin t½, 0.5–2.5 hours
 c) False   – Amiodarone t½, mean 53 (range 26–107) days
 d) True   – Gentamicin t½, 1.5–2 hours
 e) False   – Diazepam t½, 20–50 hours

11 **a)** True   It takes approximately three half-lives to reach 87.5 per cent
 b) False   of steady state. After four half-lives it is 93.75 per cent and
 c) True   after five half-lives 96.9 per cent
 d) True
 e) True

12 **a)** True   Implications of non-linear elimination kinetics include: the
 b) True   time taken to eliminate 50 per cent of a dose increases with
 c) True   increasing dose, i.e. half-life increases with dose; once the
 d) True   drug elimination process is saturated, a relatively modest
 e) False   increase in dose dramatically increases the amount of drug
 in the body see *Textbook of Clinical Pharmacology and Therapeutics*, Chapter 3

13 **a)** True   Enterohepatic circulation is when a drug is excreted into
 b) False   the bile, reabsorbed from the intestine and returned via the
 c) True   portal system to the liver to be recycled
 d) False
 e) False

14 **a)** True   See *Textbook of Clinical Pharmacology and Therapeutics*,
 b) True   Chapter 4. Although the bioavailability of two preparations
 c) True   may be the same, the kinetics can be very different as seen
 d) True   in some immediate and slow-release drug formulations
 e) True

15 **a)** True   – Levodopa → dopamine
 b) True   – Azathioprine → 6-mercaptopurine
 c) True   – Penciclovir → aciclovir
 d) True   – Sulfasalazine → aminosalicylate + sulfapyridine
 e) True   – Enalapril → enalaprilat

16 **a)** True   – Acarbose is a competitive inhibitor of intestinal
 α-glucosidases
 b) False   – Methionine, an antidote to paracematol poisoning, acts not
 in the gastrointestinal tract but predominantly in the liver
 where it repletes glutathione which inactivates the toxic
 paracetamol metabolite
 c) True   – Orlistat is used to reduce weight and is an inhibitor of
 gastrointestinal lipases and this impairs fat absorption

d) True — Olsalazine delivers 5-aminosalicylate to the colon where it has a local action in inflammatory bowel disease

e) True — Vancomycin kills toxin-producing *Clostridium difficile*, the cause of pseudomembranous colitis within the bowel

17 **a)** True Most oral drugs are absorbed by passive diffusion in the
b) False small bowel. In general low molecular weight, high lipid
c) False solubility and lack of charge encourage absorption. Most
d) True peptides are broken down enzymatically
e) False

18 **a)** False Active transport requires specific carrier-mediated energy-
b) False consuming mechanisms. Naturally occurring polar
c) True nutrients and aliments including sugars, amino acids and
d) True vitamins are absorbed by active or facilitated transport
e) True mechanisms. Drugs that are analogues of such molecules compete for uptake. Further examples include methotrexate and 5-fluorouracil

19 **a)** True Food and drink dilute the drug and can adsorb or
b) True otherwise compete with it. Transient increases in hepatic
c) False blood flow such as those that occur after a meal may result
d) False in greater availability of drug by reducing presystemic
e) False hepatic metabolism

20 **a)** False Sublingual administration can be an effective means of
b) False causing systemic effects, and has potential advantages over
c) False oral administration (i.e. when the drug is swallowed) for
d) True drugs with pronounced presystemic metabolism,
e) True providing direct and rapid access to the systemic circulation bypassing intestine and liver

21 **a)** True — Rectal indometacin administered at night is useful in reducing early morning stiffness in rheumatoid arthritis

b) False — Rectal sulfasalazine is used for its local effect in inflammatory bowel disease

c) True — Rectal metronidazole is well absorbed (and much less expensive than the intravenous preparation)

d) False — Glycerin suppositories exert a local effect to stimulate defecation

e) True — Rectal diazepam is used to control convulsions when venous access is difficult (as may be the case in children)

22 **a)** True — Transdermal GTN is used in ischaemic heart disease

b) True — Transdermal estradiol is used for hormone replacement therapy in menopausal women

c) False — Local lidocaine is used for its local anaesthetic action (e.g. for intravenous cannulation in children)

d) True   – Transcutaneous fentanyl may be administered as a patch for the treatment of chronic severe pain

e) True   – Nicotine is used to assist cigarette smokers to abstain

23 a) True   – Exercise and local massage increase the rate of absorption

b) True   – Transport from the injection site is governed by muscle blood flow – deltoid > vastus lateralis > gluteus maximus

c) True   – This avoids the risk of sciatic nerve palsy

d) False   – Up to maximum of 5 mL is acceptable in the buttock of an adult

e) True   – This depot preparation is slowly hydrolysed in muscle to release active drug and is used to improve compliance in schizophrenic patients

24 a) True   – Plus potentially fatal cardiotoxicity if rapid infusion

b) False

c) True   – An oily emulsion (Diazemuls) reduces this complication

d) True   – Used in hypoglycaemic coma but 20 per cent dextrose usually preferable

e) False

25 a) False   – Levodopa is decarboxylated to dopamine in central neurons

b) False   – Tyramine is metabolized by monoamine oxidase (MAO) in intestine, liver, kidney and nervous tissue. MAO is a mitochondrial enzyme

c) True   – Metoprolol is extensively metabolized by the CYP450 (CYP2D6) enzyme family

d) False   – Suxamethonium is metabolized by plasma cholinesterase

e) False   – Purines (e.g. 6-mercaptopurine) are metabolized by thiopurine methyl transferase and xanthine oxidase which are non-microsomal enzymes

26 a) True   – Ciclosporin is metabolized by the CYP3A family of isoenzymes

b) True   – Clarithromycin as well as being metabolized by CYP450 enzymes inhibits the metabolism of other drugs subject to CYP3A metabolism (e.g. warfarin, theophylline and terfenadine). Azithromycin does not inhibit CYP3A

c) True   – Phenytoin also induces several CYP450 enzymes

d) False   – Adrenaline is a catecholamine and is metabolized by catechol-O-methyltransferase which is present in the cytosol and MAO in mitochondria

e) True   – Warfarin has a narrow therapeutic index

27 a) True   – Dapsone is used in leprosy and dermatitis herpetiformis
    b) False – Ciclosporin, an immunosuppressant, is metabolized by
              CYP3A
    c) False – Gentamicin is eliminated unchanged by the kidney
    d) True   – Isoniazid is used to treat tuberculosis
    e) True   – Hydralazine is a vasodilator used as an adjunct to other
              treatment for hypertension. When used alone it causes
              tachycardia and fluid retention. It can cause an SLE-like
              syndrome, which is more common in slow acetylators.
              An intravenous preparation is available to treat
              hypertensive crises in pregnancy

28 a) True   – Rifampicin is a broad-spectrum antibiotic used in
              tuberculosis and Legionnaire's disease
    b) True   – Carbamazepine autoinduces its metabolism and is an
              anticonvulsant
    c) True   – St John's wort, a herbal remedy, may be purchased without
              a prescription. It is a potent, broad-spectrum CYP450
              enzyme inducer
    d) True   – Phenobarbital is an anticonvulsant
    e) False – Penicillin is predominantly eliminated unchanged in the
              urine

Drug interactions secondary to hepatic enzyme induction and inhibition are
clinically significant when there is a close correlation between plasma concentration and effect, and a steep dose response curve. Regular use of ethanol
induces CYP450 metabolism but has minimal effect on its own metabolism,
which is predominantly via cytoplasmic alcohol dehydrogenase

29 a) True   – Fluvoxamine, an antidepressant, is a selective serotonin
              reuptake inhibitor (SSRI) which inhibits the metabolism of
              theophylline and warfarin
    b) True   – Grapefruit-containing products inhibit CYP3A
              predominantly in the intestine
    c) False – Digoxin is predominantly eliminated unchanged in the
              urine
    d) True   – Itraconazole is an azole antifungal agent
    e) True   – Ciprofloxacin is a fluoroquinolone antibacterial drug

30 a) True   Presystemic metabolism occurs in the gastrointestinal
    b) False mucosa and liver; presystemic (first-pass) metabolism
    c) False necessitates high oral doses in comparison with the
    d) True   intravenous dose
    e) True

31 a) True   – Aspirin overdose decreases the rate of gastric emptying
    b) True

c) True
d) True   – Anticholinergic properties reduce gastro-intestinal motility
e) False – Metoclopramide accelerates gastric emptying

32 a) False – The absorption of thiazides is reduced
    b) False – The volume of distribution of lidocaine is reduced probably because of decreased tissue perfusion
    c) True   – The distribution volume of furosemide is largely confined to the vascular compartment
    d) False – Is prolonged predominantly due to decreased hepatic perfusion
    e) False – Glomerular filtration is reduced in cardiac failure and hence the elimination half-life of gentamicin is prolonged (i.e. not decreased)

33 a) False – Gastric pH increases
    b) True   – The ratio of unbound:bound phenytoin rises in renal failure. It is the unbound drug which is active and the laboratory assay for phenytoin measures total blood concentration (bound and unbound)
    c) True   – The blood–brain barrier becomes functionally less of a barrier to drug distribution in severe renal failure. This may be the reason for the increased incidence of confusion associated with cimetidine and famotidine in renal failure
    d) True
    e) False

34 a) True   The kidney is involved to some degree in the elimination
    b) True   of many drugs in the unchanged form and most drug
    c) True   metabolites in humans. High lipid solubility and the
    d) True   un-ionized state favour tubular reabsorption
    e) False

35 a) False
    b) False – But reduce dose; rashes more common
    c) False – May need very high doses for any diuretic effect
    d) True   – Increased risk of lactic acidosis
    e) True   – Direct nephrotoxicity, anti-anabolic, increases blood urea

36 a) True   NSAIDs cause salt and water retention and reduce renal
    b) False blood flow by inhibition of prostacyclin and prostaglandin E_2 synthesis in patients with renal compromise. This disrupts autoregulation of renal blood flow and GFR thus preventing the normal physiological mechanism which

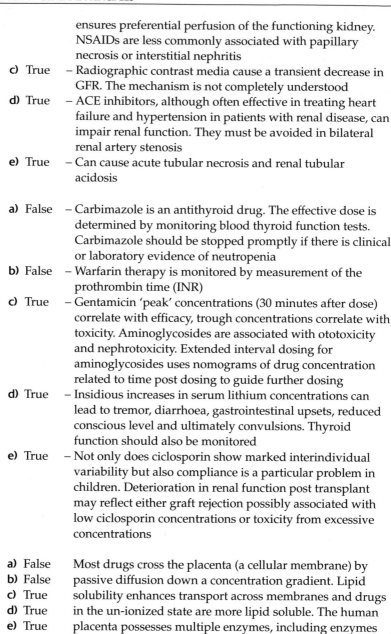

ensures preferential perfusion of the functioning kidney. NSAIDs are less commonly associated with papillary necrosis or interstitial nephritis

c) True – Radiographic contrast media cause a transient decrease in GFR. The mechanism is not completely understood

d) True – ACE inhibitors, although often effective in treating heart failure and hypertension in patients with renal disease, can impair renal function. They must be avoided in bilateral renal artery stenosis

e) True – Can cause acute tubular necrosis and renal tubular acidosis

37 a) False – Carbimazole is an antithyroid drug. The effective dose is determined by monitoring blood thyroid function tests. Carbimazole should be stopped promptly if there is clinical or laboratory evidence of neutropenia

b) False – Warfarin therapy is monitored by measurement of the prothrombin time (INR)

c) True – Gentamicin 'peak' concentrations (30 minutes after dose) correlate with efficacy, trough concentrations correlate with toxicity. Aminoglycosides are associated with ototoxicity and nephrotoxicity. Extended interval dosing for aminoglycosides uses nomograms of drug concentration related to time post dosing to guide further dosing

d) True – Insidious increases in serum lithium concentrations can lead to tremor, diarrhoea, gastrointestinal upsets, reduced conscious level and ultimately convulsions. Thyroid function should also be monitored

e) True – Not only does ciclosporin show marked interindividual variability but also compliance is a particular problem in children. Deterioration in renal function post transplant may reflect either graft rejection possibly associated with low ciclosporin concentrations or toxicity from excessive concentrations

38 a) False   Most drugs cross the placenta (a cellular membrane) by
   b) False   passive diffusion down a concentration gradient. Lipid
   c) True   solubility enhances transport across membranes and drugs
   d) True   in the un-ionized state are more lipid soluble. The human
   e) True   placenta possesses multiple enzymes, including enzymes that metabolize endogenous compounds and drugs

39 a) True – The risk of having an abnormal baby is about 10 per cent in mothers drinking 30–60 mL ethanol per day, rising to 40 per cent in chronic alcoholics

b) True   – Warfarin has been associated with nasal hypoplasia and chondrodysplasia when given in the first trimester and with CNS abnormalites and haemorrhagic complications in later pregnancy. Neonatal haemorrhage is difficult to prevent because of the immature enzymes in fetal liver and low stores of vitamin K

c) True   – All retinoic acid derivatives are teratogens. Effective contraception must be used for at least one month before, during, and at least one month after oral treatment with any retinoic acid analogue or derivative

d) False   – The minor analgesic of choice in pregnancy

e) False   – Commonly used to treat urinary tract infection in pregnancy

40   **a)** True   – This is of little consequence unless rapid drug absorption/action is required. Vomiting associated with pregnancy occasionally makes oral administration impractical

      b) True   – Blood volume in pregnancy increases by one-third

      c) True   – Plasma volume increases from 2.5 to 4 L at term and is disproportionate to the expansion in red cell mass so the haematocrit falls

      d) True   – Oedema, which at least one-third of women experience during pregnancy, may add up to 8 L to the volume of extracellular water. For water-soluble drugs (which usually have a relatively small volume of distribution) this increases the volume of distribution

      e) False   – Metabolism of drugs by the hepatocyte during pregnancy is increased

41   **a)** True   Excretion of drugs via the kidney increases because renal
      b) True   plasma flow almost doubles and the GFR increases by
      c) True   two-thirds during pregnancy, see *Textbook of Clinical*
      d) True   *Pharmacology and Therapeutics*, Chapter 9
      e) True

42   **a)** True
      b) True
      c) False   – Minimal experience, animal data discouraging
      d) False   – The fetal VIIIth nerve is more sensitive to aminoglycoside toxicity
      e) False   – Ribavirin inhibits a wide range of DNA and RNA viruses. It is used by inhalation to treat severe respiratory syncytial virus (RSV) bronchiolitis in children and is used in combination with interferon alfa to treat chronic hepatitis C infection. It is a very potent teratogen in animal models.

Effective contraception must be ensured for four months after treatment in women and seven months after treatment in men. Condoms must be used if partner of male patient (ribavirin excreted in semen) is pregnant

43 a) False   Non-drug treatment (reassurance, small frequent
    b) False   meals and advice on posture) should be pursued in the
    c) True   first instance
    d) False   – Misoprostol, an analogue of prostaglandin E_1, causes abortion
    e) True

44 a) True   – This is also true for the low molecular weight heparins (which are often the anticoagulants of choice in pregnancy)
    b) False   – Warfarin is a teratogen and is associated with a high incidence of haemorrhagic complications in late pregnancy
    c) False
    d) False
    e) False   – Pethidine, which is commonly used as an analgesic during delivery, can cause apnoea of the newborn which is reversed with naloxone

45 a) False   Epilepsy in pregnancy can lead to fetal and maternal
    b) True   morbidity/mortality through convulsions. Although all
    c) True   anticonvulsants are teratogenic, the risk of untreated
    d) True   epilepsy is greater to the mother and fetus than drug-
    e) False   induced teratogenicity. To counteract the risk of neural tube defects, adequate folate supplements are advised

46 a) False   If treatment is initiated during pregnancy it is appropriate
    b) False   to use methyldopa which has the longest record of use
    c) False   and follow-up in children born to mothers following
    d) False   treatment. Beta blockers are contraindicated in asthma.
    e) True   ACE inhibitors are teratogens. Although not licensed for use in pregnancy, nifedipine appears effective and relatively well tolerated. See *Textbook of Clinical Pharmacology and Therapeutics*, Chapter 9

47 a) False   – Commonly used to treat asthma and occasionally premature labour
    b) False   – Minimal problems when given by inhalation or in short courses (e.g. to help immature fetal lung) and although cleft palate and congenital cataract have been attributed to large systemic doses of corticosteroids the benefit of treatment usually outweighs the risk

    c) False   – Although there is an increased risk of spontaneous abortion
                  associated with general anaesthesia a causal link is unproven
                  and in most circumstances failure to operate would have
                  dramatically increased the risk to mother and fetus
    d) False   – Falciparum malaria has a high mortality in pregnancy
    e) False   – Sucralfate is not absorbed

48 a) True   Neonates are not miniature adults in terms of drug
    b) True   handling because of differences in body constitution, drug
    c) True   absorption, distribution, metabolism, excretion and
    c) True   sensitivity to adverse reactions, see *Textbook of Clinical*
    d) True   *Pharmacology and Therapeutics*, Chapter 10
    e) True

49 a) True   – Significant concentration in breast milk and there is a
                theoretical risk from iodine release
    b) False – Minimal concentration in breast milk
    c) True   – High concentration in breast milk, animal experiments
                suggest damage to growing joints
    d) True
    e) False

50 a) False – But may cause diarrhoea in infant
    b) True
    c) True
    d) False
    e) False – But gives milk an unpleasant taste

51 a) True   The total dose of drug in breast milk ingested by the
    b) True   infant is usually too small to cause problems (with some
    c) True   notable exceptions, see Table 1). The infant should be
    d) True   monitored clinically if beta-adrenoceptor antagonists
    e) False   are prescribed to the mother. Milk is mildly acid, so weak
                bases accumulate in it

52 a) True
    b) True   – A 5- to 10-day course of systemic corticosteroids is often
                sufficient
    c) False – Potentially fatal
    d) False
    e) False – Potentially fatal

53 a) True   – See *Textbook of Clinical Pharmacology and Therapeutics*,
                Chapter 11
    b) True
    c) False – One reason why plasma creatinine is a less reliable
                indicator of renal function in the elderly is that endogenous
                creatinine production is reduced

Table 1 Some drugs to be avoided during breastfeeding

Amiodarone
Aspirin
Benzodiazepines
Chloramphenicol
Ciclosporin
Ciprofloxacin
Cocaine
Combined oral contraceptives
Cytotoxics
Ergotamine
Octreotide
Stimulant laxatives (senna)
Sulfonylureas
Thiazide diuretics
Vitamin A/retinoid analogues

     d) True
     e) True

54 **a)** False   – Gliclazide, a short-acting sulfonylurea, is commonly prescribed to elderly diabetics whose blood glucose is inadequately controlled by diet alone
    b) True
    c) True   – Morphine increases bladder neck sphincter tone
    d) True   – Amitriptyline, a sedative tricyclic antidepressent, also has anticholinergic effects
    e) False

55 **a)** True   – Related to the decrease in GFR associated with ageing
    b) True   – Related to the decrease in GFR associated with ageing
    c) True   – Related to the decrease in GFR associated with ageing
    d) True   – Related to the decrease in GFR associated with ageing reducing the clearance of the active morphine glucuronide
    e) True   – Due to the increase in volume of distribution and probably also reduced metabolism

56 **a)** False
    b) False   – Finasteride is a specific inhibitor of the enzyme 5α-reductase which metabolizes testosterone into the more potent androgen, dihydrotestosterone
    c) False

d) False – Doxycycline is a unique tetracycline in that its pharmacokinetics are not affected by renal dysfunction

e) False – Has fewer anticholinergic effects than most antidepressants

57 **a)** True

b) True – Cholestatic jaundice may occur up to several weeks after treatment with flucloxacillin

c) True

d) True – Impairment of cardiovascular reflexes to erect posture in the elderly is exaggerated by alpha blockers

e) True

58 **a)** True – See *Textbook of Clinical Pharmacology and Therapeutics,* Chapter 12

b) False

c) True

d) True

e) True

59 **a)** True – Prolonged corticosteroid therapy leads to adrenal atrophy and insufficiency. Risks are minimized by the use of steroid cards, using systemic corticosteroids for the minimum period necessary and gradual withdrawal after prolonged therapy. Atrophy may persist for years after stopping corticosteroid therapy and may only be revealed during 'stress' (e.g. acute illness/surgery)

b) True – Rebound hypertension

c) True – Benzodiazepines cause psychological and physical addiction

d) True

e) False

60 **a)** False – Oral contraceptive use is associated with thromboembolism

b) True

c) True – Also associated with myocardial infarction and ischaemia to other organs

d) True

e) False – Corticosteroid therapy, if prolonged, is associated with osteoporosis. The use of antiepileptic drugs such as phenytoin and carbamazepine affect vitamin D metabolism and can lead to osteomalacia

61 **a)** True – Life-saving treatment is intramuscular adrenaline

b) False – A type II reaction

c) False – A type III reaction

d) False – A type IV reaction

e) False

62 a) True — Also associated with acne, coarse facies, hirsutism and toxic epidermal necrolysis
b) False
c) False
d) False
e) True — Usually due to the sulphamethoxazole component but may also be caused by trimethoprim

63 a) True — See *Textbook of Clinical Pharmacology and Therapeutics*, Chapter 12
b) True
c) True
d) True
e) False

64 a) True — Inactivation of penicillin
b) True — Precipitates
c) True — Precipitates
d) False
e) False

65 a) False   Approximately 45 per cent of the white population are
b) False   slow acetylators. Examples of drugs acetylated include:
c) False   isoniazid, hydralazine, phenelzine, dapsone and
d) True   procainamide. The usual 'marker' is the monoacetyl
dapsone metabolite: dapsone ratio in the plasma
e) True — Isoniazid-induced peripheral neuropathy can be prevented by prophylactic use of pyridoxine

66 a) True   The gene for G6PD is located on the X chromosome. G6PD
b) True   deficiency is more common in people from Mediterranean
c) True   countries
d) True
e) True

67 a) False   The acute porphyrias are due to hereditary enzyme defects
b) True   in haem biosynthesis and may be precipitated by many
c) True   drugs (see list in *BNF*), especially inducers of CYP450
d) True   enzymes
e) True

68 a) False   The usual response to a single intravenous dose of
b) False   suxamethonium is muscular paralysis which lasts for about
c) False   6 minutes. The effect is brief due to hydrolysis of
d) True   suxamethonium by plasma pseudocholinesterase.
e) False   Approximately 1 in 2500 patients have abnormal pseudocholinesterase which may result in prolonged paralysis for 2 hours. Inheritance is Mendelian recessive

69 a) True
   b) False – Placebo is the usual control
   c) False
   d) False
   e) False – Phase 1 studies are usually performed in healthy male
              adults aged 18–35 years

70 a) False   The MHRA is the regulatory review board of the UK who
   b) False   advise when certificates to perform clinical trials should be
   c) True   issued to pharmaceutical companies and advise, following
   d) True   review of all the data from a submission, on the granting of
   e) False   a product licence which will allow the company to market
                  the drug

71 a) True   See *Textbook of Clinical Pharmacology and Therapeutics,*
   b) True   Chapter 12
   c) True
   d) True
   e) True

72 a) True   The production of human proteins using recombinant
   b) True   DNA/RNA technology not only produces large quantities
   c) True   of natural human proteins but also minimizes the risk
   d) True   of blood-borne viral infection such as hepatitis B and C
   e) True   and HIV

EMQ ANSWERS

73 PHARMACODYNAMICS

Pharmacodynamics is the study of the effects of drugs on biological processes.

1 H Warfarin prolongs the prothrombin time and is the most commonly
   prescribed oral anticoagulant. It is a vitamin K antagonist. The onset of
   action is at least 48–72 hours after initiation of treatment following a
   loading dose. There is wide variability in drug response related to
   genetics, hepatic function, drug and alcohol interactions. Monitoring
   of treatment through measurement of INR (international normalized
   ratio) calculated from the prothrombin time is essential. Prolongation
   of INR predisposes to haemorrhage.

2 J Insulin controls the metabolic disposition of carbohydrate, fats and
   amino acids. Insulin is inactivated by gastrointestinal enzymes, hence
   administration is by injection or occasionally by inhalation. Excess
   insulin causes hypoglycaemia.

3 F Atenolol is one of the many beta-adrenoceptor blocking drugs
   available. Indications include hypertension and angina.

Beta-adrenoreceptor blockers are contraindicated in second- and third-degree heart block and asthma.

4 C Morphine, an opioid, narcotic analgesic causes pupillary constriction by stimulating μ-receptors in the Edinger–Westphal nucleus in the mid-brain. Whilst this action is not of therapeutic importance it provides a useful diagnostic sign in narcotic overdose or recent exposure.

5 A Omeprazole inhibits gastric acid secretion by blockade of the H^+/K^+ ATPase enzyme system of the gastric parietal cells. Omeprazole and other proton pump inhibitors are indicated in the management of peptic ulcers, dyspepsia and gastro-oesophageal reflux. In combination with antibacterial drugs proton pump inhibitors are used in the eradication of *Helicobacter pylori*.

74 PHARMACOKINETICS

Pharmacokinetics is defined as the study of the time-course of drug absorption, distribution, metabolism and excretion.

1 I The absorption of gentamicin (and other aminoglycoside antibacterial drugs) following oral administration is minimal. Hence gentamicin is used by injection (intramuscular and intravenous) and topically.

2 B Amiodarone, an effective antidysrhythmic drug, is only slowly eliminated by the liver, with a mean elimination half-life of 53 days. Hence effects may continue for several months after dosing has ceased.

3 E Enalapril is hydrolysed to its active metabolite, enalaprilat, which is an ACE inhibitor.

4 C Carbamazepine, an antiepileptic, induces its own metabolism such that plasma concentrations reduce significantly on repeated dosing. It has an elimination half-life of 25–60 hours following a single dose, but approximately 10 hours after repeated dosing.

5 D Lithium undergoes active tubular reabsorption. It mimics sodium on the proximal tubular sodium ion reabsorption mechanism, hence co-administration of thiazides prolongs the half-life of lithium and predisposes to toxicity.

75 PHARMACOGENETICS

Pharmacogenetics is the study of variation in drug responses under hereditary control.

1 J Approximately 70 polymorphic variants of CYP2D6 have been defined in humans. CYP2D6 enzyme is 'deficient' in about 7–10 per cent of the UK white population. Drugs affected include codeine (minimal analgesia as poor metabolizers convert little to morphine), dextrometorphan, metoprolol, some SSRIs (e.g. fluoxetine) and some antipsychotics (e.g. haloperidol).

2 **A** Drugs metabolized by CYP2C9 are eliminated more slowly by poor metabolizers who are more susceptible to dose-related adverse drug reactions (ADRs), e.g. warfarin, losartan and sulphonylureas.

3 **H** Slow and rapid acetylator status are inherited in a simple Mendelian manner, rapid metabolism is autosomal dominant. Drugs that are N-acetylated include isoniazid, dapsone, procainamide and hydralazine.

4 **G** Pseudocholinesterase hydrolyses suxamethonium, a muscle relaxant used for short procedures such as intubation since muscle paralysis lasts only 3–6 minutes. There is an autosomal recessive enzyme variant (1:2500 of the population) which is associated with prolonged paralysis requiring artificial ventilation for 2 hours or longer after an intravenous dose. Heterozygotes are unaffected.

5 **C** CYP2C19 polymorphism affects metabolism of some proton pump inhibitors e.g. omeprazole and lansoprazole. Poor metabolizers obtain greater acid suppression and improved healing rates. Other substrates for CYP2C19 include certain tricyclic and SSR1 antidepressants and R-warfarin. Warfarin is primarily a CYP2C9 substrate.

76 ABSORPTION AND ROUTE OF ADMINISTRATION

Drug absorption, and hence the route by which a particular drug may usefully be administered, is largely determined by the rate and extent of penetration of biological phospholipid membranes.

1 **I** Generic substitution seldom causes clinical problems but slow-release preparations of diltiazem, a calcium channel blocker, are an exception.

2 **B** When a drug is administered intravenously its bioavailability is by definition 100 per cent.

3 **F** Levodopa (unlike dopamine) can enter nerve terminals in the basal ganglia where it undergoes decarboxylation to form dopamine, partially correcting the nigrostriatal dopamine deficiency present in Parkinson's disease.

4 **C** Glyceryl trinitrate is used most commonly to relieve and prevent anginal pain.

5 **H** Intrathecal injection predisposes to neurotoxicity. This route should never be used without expert training.

77 DRUG METABOLISM

Drug metabolism is one of the primary mechanisms by which drugs are inactivated. However, drug metabolism in certain cases leads to increased drug activity, e.g. activation of prodrugs.

1 E Phenylephrine, an indirectly acting sympathomimetic, may cause a hypertensive crisis if taken by a patient on an MAO inhibitor.

2 C Clozapine is metabolized by CYP1A2, which is inhibited by fluvoxamine (SSRI antidepressant).

3 G Midazolam, a short-acting benzodiazepine, is often used as a 'probe' in studies to determine if a drug induces or inhibits CYP3A4 metabolism.

4 B Patients with Gilbert's disease have unconjugated hyperbilirubinaemia caused by an inherited deficiency of UGT1AI. Fasting and oestrogens may aggravate jaundice. Gilbert's disease is almost always irrelevant to drug metabolism with the exception of the active metabolite of irinotecan (used in metastatic colon cancer), whose toxicity is increased in Gilbert's disease.

5 A 6-Mercaptopurine (6-MP) is the active metabolite of azathioprine. Bone marrow suppression is more likely in those deficient in thiopurine methyltransferase (0.3 per cent of white population).

78 RENAL ELIMINATION

The kidneys are involved in the elimination of virtually every drug or drug metabolite.

1 G Gentamicin, an aminoglycoside antibacterial drug with a low therapeutic index, is predominantly eliminated via the kidney.

2 C Probenecid competes for the proximal tubule active secretion of organic anions hence reduces the tubular secretion of penicillin and methotrexate.

3 D Urinary alkalinization enhances the excretion of salicylate reducing toxicity after salicylate/aspirin overdose.

4 F Hence salt depletion which causes increased proximal tubular sodium ion reabsorption causes lithium toxicity unless the dose of lithium is reduced.

5 B Para-aminohippuric acid is excreted so efficiently that it is completely extracted from the renal plasma in a single pass through the kidney.

79 RENAL TRACT

1 F Acetazolamide is a carbonic anhydrase inhibitor that reduces aqueous humour production which is beneficial in glaucoma. It is a weak diuretic and has a specific role in treating epilepsy associated with menstruation.

2 E Spironolactone's active metabolite, canrenone, is an aldosterone antagonist, which also acts on sex hormone receptors and can cause gynaecomastia, menstrual disorders and testicular atrophy.

3 G Bendroflumethiazide blocks tubular Na^+/Cl^- reabsorption.

4 C Furosemide and other loop diuretics enhance aminoglycoside ototoxicity through their action on $Na^+/K^+/2Cl^-$ co-transport in the inner ear.

5 A Sildenafil inhibits phosphodiesterase V that inactivates cGMP; glyceryl trinitrate activates guanylate cyclase and the combination can cause severe hypotension.

80 ADVERSE DRUG REACTIONS

Adverse drug reactions are unwanted effects caused by normal therapeutic doses of drugs.

1 G Spironolactone acts as a potassium-sparing diuretic through its antagonism of aldosterone, but also acts on progesterone and androgen receptors.

2 D Osteoporosis is an important adverse effect with chronic use of prednisolone and all other glucocorticosteroids (diabetes is another).

3 C Myositis is a dose-related adverse effect associated with statins and fibrates.

4 F SLE-like syndrome is associated with isoniazid, procainamide, hydralazine, chlorpromazine and anticonvulsants. It resembles SLE together with a positive antinuclear factor test. It is dose related. These drugs may act as haptens, combining with DNA and forming antigens. The symptoms resolve (sometimes slowly) on drug withdrawal.

5 J Tardive dyskinesia is a troublesome adverse effect associated predominantly with 'traditional' D_2-blocking antipsychotic drugs, which follows months or years of continued treatment.

81 MONOCLONAL ANTIBODIES

Monoclonal antibodies are highly specific antibodies derived from one class of cells which recognize one antigen. Receptor affinity is high and toxicity is likely to be due to exaggerated pharmacological action or hypersensitivity.

1 J Palivizumab (Synagis®) is used in 'at-risk' infants to prevent serious lower respiratory-tract disease caused by RSV. At-risk infants includes those with serious congenital heart disease.

2 G Omalizumab (Xolair®) binds to IgE and can be used as additional therapy in asthmatics with proven IgE sensitivity to inhaled allergens whose asthma is inadequately controlled by high-dose glucocorticosteroids (systemic and inhaled); optimal bronchodilator therapy (short- and long-acting beta-2 agonists plus anticholinergics) plus oral leukotriene antagonists.

3 A Infliximab (Remicade®) inhibits TNF activity and is used in rheumatoid arthritis and psoriatic arthritis in adults who have failed to respond to at least two other disease-modifying agents (e.g. penicillamine and methotrexate). It can also be used in inflammatory bowel disease.

4 B Bevacizumab (Avastin®) inhibits VEGF. It is a first-line treatment for metastatic colorectal cancer in combination with 5 fluorouracil plus folinic acid plus irinotecan (FOLFIRI).

5 F Abciximab (ReoPro®) binds to platelet IIb/IIIa receptors blocking fibrinogen binding. It is used as an adjunct to heparin and aspirin in high-risk patients undergoing percutaneous coronary intervention. It can be used once only to avoid thrombocytopenia.

CHAPTER TWO

NERVOUS SYSTEM

MULTIPLE CHOICE QUESTIONS

82 Benzodiazepines:
  a) Potentiate the sedative effects of alcohol
  b) Should only be used as hypnotics for a maximum of 2–4 weeks
  c) Suppress rapid eye movement (REM) sleep
  d) Act by binding to the gamma-aminobutyric acid (GABA) receptor–chloride channel complex and facilitate the opening of the channel in the presence of GABA
  e) Are anxiolytic

83 Benzodiazepine dependence and withdrawal syndrome:
  a) Benzodiazepine withdrawal symptoms should be treated with buspirone
  b) Fits can occur in the first week after withdrawal
  c) The full withdrawal picture usually appears after an interval of 3–8 weeks
  d) Perceptual distortions are characteristic
  e) Shorter-acting benzodiazepines are less likely to cause dependence and should be substituted for long-acting benzodiazepines when withdrawing a patient from benzodiazepines

84 Diazepam:
  a) Has a half-life of less than 20 hours
  b) Can cause anterograde amnesia
  c) Is effective in terminating acute dystonia caused by metoclopramide
  d) Never causes fatal overdose
  e) The major site of metabolism is the liver

85 Temazepam:
  a) Has a shorter half-life than diazepam
  b) Potentiates the effects of alcohol
  c) Causes no 'hangover' effect 10 hours post dosing
  d) Is not addictive
  e) Is more potent than lorazepam

86 Clomethiazole (chlormethiazole):

a) Is not absorbed orally
b) Has a half-life of approximately 10 hours
c) In cirrhosis the bioavailability is increased about 10-fold
d) High doses cause cardiovascular and respiratory depression
e) Is antagonized by ethanol

87 Promethazine:

a) Is a GABA agonist
b) Is available without prescription
c) Causes dry mouth, constipation and reduced sweating
d) Liver failure is an absolute contraindication
e) May cause hallucinations

88 Zopiclone:

a) Is an ultra short-acting benzodiazepine
b) Is the hypnotic of choice in a breastfeeding mother
c) Is a more effective anticonvulsant than clonazepam
d) Is associated with drug dependence
e) Can cause confusion

89 The following drugs may mimic some of the common clinical features of schizophrenia:

a) Levodopa
b) Salbutamol
c) LSD
d) Diamorphine
e) Methylenedioxymethylamphetamine (MDMA, ecstasy)

90 Blockade of central D_2 receptors:

a) Parallels the clinical efficacy of the conventional antipsychotic drugs such as chlorpromazine and haloperidol
b) Induces extrapyramidal effects
c) Repeated administration of D_2 antagonists causes a reduction in D_2 agonist sensitivity due to an increase in abundance of these receptors
d) Repeated administration of D_2 antagonists may lead to tardive dyskinesia
e) Causes a decrease in cardiac output

91 Adverse effects associated with phenothiazines include:

a) Dry mouth
b) Blurred vision
c) Postural hypotension
d) Impaired temperature control
e) Jaundice

92 Chlorpromazine:

a) Is the first-line treatment for malignant neuroleptic syndrome

b) Has a low volume of distribution (approx. 100 mL/kg)

c) Is predominantly eliminated via the kidneys as unchanged chlorpromazine

d) Of the chlorpromazine in plasma, 90–95 per cent is bound to plasma proteins

e) Usually once-daily administration is adequate

93 Flupentixol:

a) Is particularly effective in mania

b) May be given once every 2–4 weeks via the intramuscular route for chronic schizophrenia

c) Is less sedating than chlorpromazine

d) Is more prone than chlorpromazine to produce extrapyramidal toxicity

e) Should not be used in patients with porphyria

94 Clozapine:

a) Has weak D_2-blocking activity

b) Is effective in up to 60 per cent of patients who have not responded to phenothiazines

c) Is effective against negative as well as positive symptoms

d) Rarely causes tardive dyskinesia

e) Causes blood dyscrasias more commonly than most antipsychotics

95 Newer atypical drugs such as olanzapine and risperidone:

a) Are less effective than traditional antipsychotic drugs against the negative symptoms of schizophrenia

b) Are associated with weight loss

c) Bind irreversibly to D_2 receptors

d) Are associated with an increased incidence of stroke in elderly patients with dementia

e) Are virtually free from extrapyramidal side-effects at standard doses

96 The following drugs raise synaptic and/or total brain monoamines:

a) Cocaine

b) Amitriptyline

c) Imipramine

d) Phenelzine

e) Amphetamine

97 Tricyclic antidepressants:

a) Are more effective in endogenous rather than reactive depression
b) Are particularly effective when the depression is associated with psychomotor and physiological changes
c) Onset of therapeutic action is approximately two weeks after starting therapy
d) Are effective in the management of panic disorder
e) Are used for the treatment of nocturnal enuresis in children

98 Antidepressants with sedative properties include:

a) Amitriptyline
b) Dosulepin
c) Citalopram
d) Paroxetine
e) Sertraline

99 The following are consistent with tricyclic antidepressant overdose:

a) Dilated pupils
b) Hyperreflexia
c) Sinus tachycardia
d) Widened QRS on the ECG
e) Convulsions

100 Amitriptyline:

a) Is highly lipid soluble
b) Is highly protein bound
c) Has a low volume of distribution (approx. 100 mL/kg body weight)
d) Blocks uptake of monoamines into cerebral and other neurons
e) Delays gastric emptying

101 Fluvoxamine:

a) Inhibits monoamine oxidase (MAO)
b) Is a powerful anticholinergic agent
c) Is less sedative than trazodone
d) Inhibits a CYP450 isoenzyme
e) During therapy the blood count should be monitored weekly

102 Fluoxetine:

a) Selectively blocks neuronal uptake of noradrenaline
b) Is more cardiotoxic than imipramine
c) Is less sedative than amitriptyline
d) Is associated with nausea and dyspepsia
e) Has a short elimination half-life of 1–2 hours

103 Phenelzine:
   a) Is a reversible selective inhibitor of MAO-B
   b) Onset of therapeutic effect is usually within one week
   c) Is ineffective if used alone in the treatment of depression
   d) Is sometimes effective in reducing hypochondriacal and hysterical symptoms
   e) Is more likely to cause a hypertensive crisis when an indirectly acting sympathomimetic (e.g. ephedrine) is given concurrently rather than a directly acting sympathomimetic (e.g. adrenaline combined with local anaesthetic)

104 Moclobemide:
   a) Is a reversible selective inhibitor of MAO-A
   b) Is effective adjunct therapy in Parkinson's disease
   c) Has a longer duration of MAO inhibition compared to phenelzine after stopping therapy
   d) Causes dry mouth in over 50 per cent of patients
   e) Is less likely than phenelzine to cause a food (tyramine) interaction

105 The following foodstuffs can cause a hypertensive/hyperthermic reaction during non-selective MAO inhibitor therapy:
   a) Cheese
   b) Yoghurt
   c) Beer
   d) Marmite
   e) Grouse

106 Lithium toxicity can be precipitated by:
   a) Sodium depletion
   b) Thiazide therapy
   c) Angiotensin-converting enzyme (ACE) inhibitors
   d) Non-steroidal anti-inflammatory drugs (NSAIDs)
   e) Atenolol

107 Tricyclic antidepressant therapy should not be started within 14 days of therapy with:
   a) Citalopram
   b) Isocarboxazid
   c) Tranylcypromine
   d) Moclobemide
   e) St John's wort

108 Muscarinic antagonists (e.g. procyclidine):

a) Are predominantly used in parkinsonism caused by antipsychotic drugs
b) Are least effective in the treatment of tremor
c) Are ineffective in the management of post-encephalitic parkinsonism
d) Must not be used with levodopa
e) May cause confusion in the elderly

109 The following enhance central dopaminergic activity:

a) Inhibition of MAO-B
b) Bromocriptine
c) Apomorphine
d) Haloperidol
e) Intravenous dopamine

110 Levodopa:

a) Can enter nerve terminals
b) Is oxidized by MAO to form dopamine
c) Is antagonized by ropinirole
d) Metabolism is reduced by entacapone
e) May cause dystonic reactions

111 Levodopa:

a) Is the amino acid precursor of dopamine
b) Improves bradykinesia and rigidity more than tremor
c) Levodopa therapy should be initiated with a loading dose
d) Should be taken on an empty stomach
e) Involuntary movements and psychiatric complications are common unwanted effects

112 Bromocriptine:

a) Stimulates release of endogenous dopamine
b) Stimulates postsynaptic D_2 receptors
c) Should not be prescribed until there is inadequate response to levodopa
d) Has an antiemetic action
e) Inhibits the release of prolactin from the pituitary

113 Selegiline:

a) Selectively inhibits MAO-B
b) The most common adverse effect is postural hypotension
c) Is principally eliminated unchanged in the urine
d) Cannot be prescribed concurrently with levodopa
e) Cannot be prescribed concurrently with amantadine

114 The following drugs reduce spasticity in patients with upper motor neuron lesions:
- **a)** Donepezil
- **b)** Riluzole
- **c)** Diazepam
- **d)** Baclofen
- **e)** Dantrolene

115 Tardive dyskinesia:
- **a)** Occurs in about 15 per cent of patients treated with phenothiazines for over 2 years
- **b)** Stopping treatment results in slow improvement in approximately 40 per cent of patients
- **c)** Dyskinesia may initially worsen after discontinuing treatment
- **d)** Consists of rapid involuntary movements of the limbs
- **e)** Is treated with botulinum toxin A

116 In myasthenia gravis:
- **a)** Therapy is usually initiated with neostigmine
- **b)** Thymectomy may be beneficial
- **c)** Corticosteroids and azathioprine reduce circulating T cells
- **d)** There is increased sensitivity to atenolol
- **e)** Corticosteroids can worsen or improve weakness

117 Severe weakness in a patient with myasthenia gravis may be potentiated by:
- **a)** Spontaneous deterioration in the natural history of the disease
- **b)** Excessive anticholinesterase drug
- **c)** Acute infection
- **d)** Aminoglycosides
- **e)** Fluoxetine

118 In Alzheimer's disease:
- **a)** Donepezil can slow down the progression of mild and moderate Alzheimer's disease
- **b)** Rivastigmine acts through reversible inhibition of acetylcholinesterase
- **c)** Adverse effects associated with donepezil, rivastigmine and galantamine include nausea, vomiting and diarrhoea
- **d)** Overdose with donepezil is likely to be associated with tachycardia
- **e)** Associated depression may be treated with a selective serotonin reuptake inhibitor

119 The following drugs are effective in partial seizures with or without secondary generalized tonic clonic seizures:
   a) Carbamazepine
   b) Valproate
   c) Topiramate
   d) Lamotrigine
   e) Ethosuximide

120 The following adverse effects are associated with sodium valproate therapy:
   a) Tremor
   b) Nausea, vomiting and abdominal pain
   c) Ventricular tachycardia
   d) Thrombocytosis
   e) Hair loss (temporary)

121 The following are recognized adverse effects associated with phenytoin therapy:
   a) Ataxia
   b) Dysarthria
   c) Acne
   d) Hyperkalaemia
   e) Macrocytic anaemia

122 The pharmacokinetics of phenytoin are characterized by:
   a) Wide interindividual variation
   b) Less than 10 per cent systemic bioavailability if taken by mouth with food
   c) Two populations – fast and slow acetylators
   d) The half-life is not affected by dose
   e) Once-daily dosing is adequate

123 Carbamazepine:
   a) Inhibits GABA transaminase
   b) Inhibits its own metabolism
   c) Is effective in temporal lobe epilepsy
   d) Inhibits the metabolism of warfarin
   e) Modified-release tablets significantly lessen the incidence of dose-related side-effects

124 The following adverse effects are associated with carbamazepine therapy:
   a) Trigeminal neuralgia
   b) Sedation
   c) Dizziness
   d) Diplopia
   e) Hyponatraemia

125 Sodium valproate:

  a) Is a dopamine antagonist

  b) Is indicated in tonic–clonic epilepsy

  c) Blood concentration should be monitored frequently during treatment

  d) Rarely causes hepatic necrosis

  e) Is safe in pregnancy

126 Vigabatrin:

  a) Is a structural analogue of GABA

  b) Increases the brain concentration of GABA

  c) Can cause visual field defects

  d) May cause hallucinations and paranoia

  e) Is excreted unchanged in bile

127 The following antiepileptics induce the metabolism of oestrogen and can lead to unwanted pregnancies in women using oral contraception:

  a) Carbamazepine

  b) Phenytoin

  c) Sodium valproate

  d) Phenobarbital

  e) Lamotrigine

128 An 18-year-old man is admitted to casualty in status epilepticus. There is a history of three previous unexplained blackouts in the last year. The following are appropriate:

  a) Intravenous lorazepam

  b) Intramuscular phenytoin

  c) Measurement of blood glucose

  d) Administration of 24 per cent oxygen

  e) Once the acute episode is over oral gabapentin should be commenced

129 Febrile convulsions:

  a) Approximately 3 per cent of children have at least one febrile convulsion

  b) A prolonged convulsion can usually be terminated with rectal diazepam

  c) Paracetamol is contraindicated in children who have febrile convulsions

  d) Regular prophylaxis with phenobarbital reduces the likelihood of adult epilepsy

  e) Children with recurrent febrile convulsions should take prophylactic penicillin

130   In acute migraine the following are correct:

   a) Paracetamol NSAID or aspirin is usually the treatment of choice
   b) Metoclopramide may be effective due to its dopamine agonist action
   c) Ergotamine may be given by the rectal route
   d) Sumatriptan probably works through its $5HT_{1D}$ agonist properties
   e) Pizotifen is effective when given by intramuscular injection during the acute episode

131   Sumatriptan:

   a) Has a greater bioavailability after subcutaneous injection than oral administration
   b) Is contraindicated in patients with ischaemic heart disease
   c) Causes a significant, but transient, pressor response
   d) Should not be combined with ergotamine
   e) Metabolism is inhibited by paracetamol

132   The following are used in the prophylaxis of migraine:

   a) Rizatriptan
   b) Ergotamine
   c) Pizotifen
   d) Propranolol
   e) Methysergide

133   In comparison to halothane, sevoflurane:

   a) Is associated with more rapid recovery
   b) Is more likely to cause hepatic necrosis
   c) Is less likely to cause ventricular dysrhythmias
   d) Is more extensively metabolized by the liver
   e) Is more expensive

134   Fentanyl:

   a) Has powerful analgesic properties
   b) Is a powerful muscle relaxant
   c) Acts within 1–2 minutes following intravenous administration
   d) Undergoes rapid metabolism by non-specific blood and tissue esterases
   e) To avoid excessive dosage in obese patients dose may need to be calculated on the basis of ideal body weight

135   Nitrous oxide:

   a) Is a powerful muscle relaxant
   b) Is predominantly excreted by exhalation
   c) During recovery transient hypoxia may occur in patients with respiratory disease
   d) Increases blood pressure and heart rate
   e) Is antagonized by naloxone

136 Propofol in comparison to thiopental sodium:

a) Cannot be used for induction of anaesthesia
b) Has a longer elimination half-life
c) Has no active metabolites
d) Is less irritant
e) Produces a more rapid 'clear headed' recovery

137 The following agents may be used as premedication for anaesthesia:

a) Hyoscine
b) Temazepam
c) Morphine
d) Neostigmine
e) Ketamine

138 Atracurium:

a) Is a non-depolarizing muscle relaxant
b) Has histamine-blocking properties
c) May be used as a continuous infusion in intensive care to facilitate intermittent positive pressure ventilation
d) Is metabolized in the liver
e) Patients with reduced renal function show reduced elimination and prolonged neuromuscular blockade

139 The following would be suitable for postoperative analgesia in a patient with severe chronic obstructive airways disease with CO_2 retention who has had an abdominoperineal resection:

a) Intramuscular morphine
b) Epidural block with bupivacaine
c) Rectal diclofenac
d) Intramuscular diclofenac
e) Oral oxycodone

140 The following are indicated in the management of malignant hyperthermia due to volatile anaesthetics or suxamethonium:

a) Discontinuation of anaesthetic
b) 100 per cent oxygen
c) Intravenous dantrolene
d) Correction of acidosis and hyperkalaemia
e) Cooling

141 Lidocaine, a local anaesthetic:

a) Prevents the rapid inflow of sodium ions which is the ionic basis of the action potential
b) Causes vasoconstriction
c) Is not absorbed from the urethra
d) Can be combined with adrenaline for digital 'ring' blocks
e) Has a shorter duration of action than bupivacaine

142 The following drugs are correctly paired with their putative site(s) of action:

a) NSAIDs – at the site of injury, by interfering with the chemical mediators involved in nociception
b) Paracetamol – peripheral inhibition of cyclo-oxygenase
c) Lidocaine – block of transmission in peripheral nerves
d) Opioids – modification of transmission at the dorsal horn
e) Opioids – interference with central appreciation of pain and inhibition of emotional concomitants

143 Aspirin:

a) Inhibits cyclo-oxygenase irreversibly
b) Produces its major analgesic and anti-inflammatory effects by inhibition of prostaglandin E_2 and prostacyclin biosynthesis
c) Impairs colour vision
d) Acts on the hypothalamus to reduce body temperature
e) Chronic use is associated with iron-deficiency anaemia

144 Adverse effects associated with salicylates include:

a) Claudication
b) Bronchoconstriction
c) Systemic lupus erythematosus
d) Hepatitis
e) Reye's syndrome

145 Ibuprofen:

a) Is a reversible cyclo-oxygenase inhibitor
b) Has analgesic properties
c) Has antipyretic properties
d) Has anti-inflammatory properties
e) Can cause renal impairment

146 Nefopam:

a) Is associated with gastrointestinal haemorrhage
b) Causes miosis
c) Causes more respiratory depression than morphine
d) Potentiates the dysrhythmogenic effect of halothane anaesthesia
e) Is contraindicated in epilepsy

147 Co-codamol contains:

a) Aspirin
b) Paracetamol
c) Dextropropoxyphene
d) Caffeine
e) Promethazine

148 Morphine:

a) Acts as an agonist at opioid receptors (especially μ) in the brain and spinal cord
b) Causes pupillary constriction by stimulation of the Edinger–Westphal nucleus in the mid-brain
c) Acts as an antihistamine
d) Is subject to presystemic metabolism
e) Stimulates the chemoreceptor trigger zone

149 The following are particularly sensitive to the pharmacological actions of morphine:

a) Young children
b) The elderly
c) Patients with hepatic failure
d) Patients with renal failure
e) Patients with hyperthyroidism

150 Morphine causes:

a) Diarrhoea
b) Increased intrabiliary pressure
c) Histamine release
d) Reduced sensitivity of the respiratory centre to carbon dioxide
e) Vasoconstriction

151 Pethidine:

a) Is more potent than morphine
b) Does not cause respiratory depression
c) Always causes pupillary constriction at analgesic doses
d) Suppresses cough at analgesic doses
e) Reduces the activity of the pregnant term uterus

152 Codeine:

a) Is a metabolite of morphine
b) Has a plasma half-life of approximately 12 hours
c) Its effects are antagonized by naloxone
d) Is used as a cough suppressant
e) Causes constipation

153 Buprenorphine:

a) Is a partial agonist on opioid receptors
b) Occupies a much larger fraction of opioid receptors to produce its analgesic effect than does morphine
c) Should only be used to treat acute pain
d) Is subject to prescription requirements under the Misuse of Drugs Act
e) May be administered sublingually

154 Naloxone:

a) Binds to opioid μ receptors
b) Acts as a partial opioid agonist
c) Has little effect on a healthy person who has not taken opioid drugs
d) Has an elimination half-life of approximately 12 hours
e) Is contraindicated in young children

Answers: see pages 55–66

EXTENDED MATCHING QUESTIONS

155 CENTRALLY ACTIVE DRUGS

A	Temazepam	F	Orphenadrine
B	Lithium	G	Sumatriptan
C	Citalopram	H	Aripiprazole
D	Haloperidol	I	Gabapentin
E	Pizotifen	J	Valproate

For each clinical scenario below, suggest the most appropriate therapy:

1   Acute migraine in a 20-year-old woman, which is unresponsive to paracetamol, ibuprofen and metoclopramide
2   A 40-year-old man with troublesome myoclonic jerks
3   A 70-year-old man with schizophrenia, who has developed incapacitating tardive dyskinesia on his maintenance therapy of oral chlorpromazine
4   A 40-year-old man with endogenous depression
5   Severe disabling insomnia

156 DRUG-INDUCED MOVEMENT DISORDERS

A	Interferon beta	F	Esmolol
B	Ciprofloxacin	G	Prednisolone
C	Salbutamol	H	Pioglitazone
D	Doxazosin	I	Phenytoin
E	Gentamicin	J	Ranitidine

Select the drug from the list above that is most likely to be the cause of the effect below:

1   Tremor
2   'Cerebellar' ataxia
3   Vestibular toxicity causing loss of balance
4   Proximal myopathy
5   Tenosynovitis

157 TREATMENT OF MOVEMENT DISORDERS AND DEMENTIA

A	Botulinum toxin	**F**	Zopiclone
B	Procyclidine	**G**	Ropinirole
C	Donepezil	**H**	Buspirone
D	Phenelzine	**I**	Thiamine
E	Lamotrigine	**J**	Neostigmine

Select the drug from the above list which is licensed for the indication below:

1 Idiopathic Parkinson's disease
2 Hemifacial spasm
3 Myasthenia
4 Fluphenazine-induced dystonia
5 Alzheimer's disease

158 ANALGESICS/PAIN

A	Fentanyl	**F**	Indometacin
B	Aspirin	**G**	Morphine
C	Nefopam	**H**	Paracetamol
D	Allopurinol	**I**	Metoclopramide
E	Pregabalin	**J**	Ephedrine

Link each of 1 to 5 below with the most appropriate item from A to J:

1 Mild analgesic suitable for children
2 Suitable for acute gout
3 Used by injection for patient-controlled self-administration
4 Overdose causes tinnitus
5 Can be administered as transdermal patch

ANSWERS: see pages 66–68

ANSWERS

MCQ ANSWERS

82 **a)** True   Benzodiazepines, whilst being much safer than the
    b) True   barbiturates, still have the problems of dependence,
    c) True   potentiation of alcohol, respiratory depression in overdose
    d) True   and suppressing REM sleep
    e) True

83 **a)** False   – Buspirone is a non-benzodiazepine anxiolytic drug. It does
                 not have marked hypnotic, anticonvulsant or muscle
                 relaxant properties. It does not alleviate benzodiazepine
                 withdrawal symptoms
    b) True
    c) False   – The full withdrawal picture usually appears after an
                 interval of 3–8 days
    d) True
    e) False   – It is common practice to substitute shorter-acting with
                 longer-acting benzodiazepines (e.g. temazepam to
                 diazepam) to assist withdrawal

84 **a)** False   – Up to 50 hours, the active desmethyl metabolite has a half-
                 life of 36–200 hours
    b) True
    c) True
    d) False   – Usually in combination with alcohol or other drugs
    e) True

85 **a)** True   – 5–6 hours in comparison with 20–50 hours
    b) True   – This combination is a cause of fatal overdose as well as
                 disinhibited behaviour which may lead to crime or road
                 traffic accidents
    c) False   – Patients must be warned not to drive or operate heavy
                 machinery if affected
    d) False   – Temazepam is a controlled drug
    e) False

86 **a)** False   – Absorption is rapid with peak plasma levels being
                 obtained at 60 minutes. Clomethiazole undergoes extensive
                 first-pass metabolism so oral bioavailability is only
                 approximately 15 per cent
    b) False   – The half-life is 50 minutes. The short half-life reduces the
                 risk of hangover, ataxia and confusion the next day
    c) True   – This results from decreased first-pass metabolism

56 CHAPTER 2 NERVOUS SYSTEM

d) True   – Fatalities have occurred because of poorly supervised intravenous infusions. Constant rate infusions lead to accumulation

e) False   – It potentiates the effects of alcohol although it may be used to treat acute alcohol withdrawal

87   **a)** False   – Promethazine is an H_1 antihistamine
     b) True
     c) True   – Antimuscarinic effects
     d) True   – May cause coma
     e) True

88   **a)** False   Zopiclone is a non-benzodiazepine hypnotic which enhances
     b) False   GABA activity. In addition to sedation adverse effects include
     c) False   bitter, metallic taste, anorexia, nausea and vomiting, visual
     d) True   hallucinations, amnesia, aggression and agitation
     e) True

89   **a)** True   Occasionally drug-induced hallucinations/psychosis may
     b) False   be mistaken for schizophrenia. The hypothesis that chronic
     c) True   cannabis use and LSD can cause schizophrenia is unproven
     d) False
     e) True

90   **a)** True   Prolonged use of D_2 receptor blockers is associated with
     b) True   the onset of tardive dyskinesia which may involve
     c) False   structural brain damage and is often irreversible
     d) True
     e) False

91   **a)** True   – Anticholinergic
     b) True   – Anticholinergic
     c) True   – Peripheral alpha-adrenoceptor blockade
     d) True   – Hypothermia in cold weather, hyperthermia in hot weather
     e) True   – Jaundice occurs in 0.5 per cent of patients taking chlorpromazine. It is due to intrahepatic cholestasis and is a hypersensitivity phenomenon associated with eosinophilia

92   **a)** False   – Antipsychotic drugs may cause maligant neuroleptic syndrome. This rare syndrome (hyperthermia, varying conscious level, rigidity and autonomic dysfunction) may be treated with dantrolene or bromocriptine
     b) False   – Volume of distribution is large, approximately 22 L/kg
     c) False   – Metabolism predominantly by hepatic microsomes. Over 70 metabolites have been identified
     d) True
     e) True

93 a) False   Depot intramuscular preparations such as flupentixol
       b) True   decanoate are valuable in the management of
       c) True   schizophrenia for maintenance therapy to ensure
       d) True   compliance which is often poor in such patients
       e) True

94 a) True   Clozapine is an 'atypical antipsychotic'. The term is used
       b) True   imprecisely but generally covers those antipsychotic drugs
       c) True   whose principal pharmacological effect is not D_2 blockade
       d) True   and are rarely associated with extrapyramidal side-effects
       e) True   – Neutropenia or agranulocytosis develops in up to 3 per
                    cent of patients taking clozapine for 1 year. Although
                    dystonias and tardive dyskinesias are rare, clozapine is
                    associated with fits in 3–4 per cent of patients and postural
                    hypotension (particularly after the first dose)

95 a) False   In comparison to the conventional antipsychotics where
       b) False   potency is closely related to D_2 receptor blockade, atypical
       c) False   antipsychotics bind less tightly to D_2 receptors and have
       d) True   additional pharmacological activity which varies with the
       e) True   drug. Efficacy against negative symptoms as well as fewer
                    extrapyramidal side-effects are characteristic. These may be
                    the result of the transient ('hit and run') binding to D_2
                    receptors. May also block D_4 and $5HT_2$ receptors

96 a) True   Tricyclic drugs of the amitriptyline type raise synaptic
       b) True   stores of NA and 5HT and are antidepressant. MAO
       c) True   inhibitors which increase total brain NA and 5HT are also
       d) True   antidepressant. Amphetamine and cocaine raise synaptic
       e) True   NA and alter mood but are not antidepressant

97 a) True   See *Textbook of Clinical Pharmacology and Therapeutics*,
       b) True   Chapter 20. Although clinical experience is most
       c) True   extensive with the tricyclic antidepressants, the side-effect
       d) True   profile of selective serotonin reuptake inhibitors (SSRIs) is
       e) True   usually less troublesome and these drugs are safer in
                    overdose

98 a) True   The less sedative tricyclic and related antidepressants
       b) True   include desipramine, imipramine, lofepramine and
       c) False   nortriptyline. Protriptyline is a stimulant. The more
       d) False   sedative drugs are preferred for agitated and anxious
       e) False   patients, whilst the less sedative are preferred in
                    withdrawn patients. Citalopram, paroxetine and
                    sertraline are SSRIs. SSRIs are less sedating than most
                    tricyclic antidepressants. Insomnia occurs in some
                    patients on SSRIs

99 a) True   Tricyclic antidepressant overdoses are commonly fatal.
b) True   Patients may die from cardiac dysrhythmias, convulsions or
c) True   direct CNS depression leading to respiratory arrest/
d) True   asphyxia. See *Textbook of Clinical Pharmacology and*
e) True   *Therapeutics*, Chapter 54

100 a) True   Amitriptyline is a sedative tricyclic antidepressant which is
b) True   usually administered as a single nocte dose
c) False
d) True
e) True

101 a) False   – Fluvoxamine is an SSRI
b) False
c) True
d) True   – Fluvoxamine inhibits CYP1A2 and therefore decreases the
metabolism of theophylline and warfarin. Both these drugs
have a narrow therapeutic index hence their concomitant
administration with fluvoxamine should be avoided if
possible
e) False

102 a) False   Fluoxetine is an SSRI. It is safer in overdose and causes
b) False   fewer antimuscarinic side-effects than the tricyclic
c) True   antidepressants. The most common adverse effects related
d) True   to SSRIs are nausea, dyspepsia, diarrhoea, dry mouth,
e) False   headache, insomnia and dizziness. Sweating, erectile
dysfunction and delayed orgasm are well-recognized
associations

103 a) False   Phenelzine (and isocarboxazid and tranylcypromine) are
b) False   irreversible non-selective MAO inhibitors
c) False
d) True
e) True   – Adrenaline is metabolized by catechol-O-methyltransferase

104 a) True   – Moclobemide is a reversible, competitive, selective MAO-A
inhibitor
b) False   – Selegiline, an MAO-B inhibitor, is used in Parkinson's disease
c) False
d) False   – No anticholinergic action (cf. tricyclic antidepressants)
e) True

105 a) True   Patients on MAO inhibitors should be given a treatment
b) True   card which lists necessary precautions. Interactions with
c) True   foodstuffs, many proprietary preparations and prescribed
d) True   drugs may cause a hypertensive crisis. Phenotolamine
e) True   and/or labetalol are effective treatment for such a reaction

106 a) True   Lithium salts have a narrow therapeutic index. Lithium
    b) True   concentrations may rise insidiously and once adverse
    c) True   effects such as tremor, ataxia, dysarthria and nystagmus
    d) True   develop treatment must be stopped whilst the serum
    e) False   lithium (avoid lithium heparin tubes to collect plasma) is
                    measured urgently

107 a) False   – Selective serotonin reuptake inhibitor
    b) True   – Irreversible non-selective MAO inhibitor
    c) True   – Irreversible non-selective MAO inhibitor
    d) False   – Reversible selective MAO inhibitor
    e) False   – St John's wort is a herbal remedy which is popular for self-treatment of depression. It is a potent CYP450 enzyme inducer

108 a) True   Muscarinic antagonists are effective in the treatment of
    b) False   parkinsonian tremor and to a lesser extent rigidity. They
    c) False   have minimal effects on bradykinesia. Although more
    d) False   commonly prescribed to counteract antipsychotic drug-
    e) True   induced parkinsonism they may be used alone in idiopathic parkinsonism and postencephalitic parkinsonism if tremor is the predominant symptom

109 a) True   Parkinsonism arises because of deficient dopaminergic
    b) True   transmission. Bromocriptine and apomorphine are
    c) True   dopamine receptor agonists. Acetylcholine is antagonistic
    d) False   to dopamine within the striatum
    e) False

110 a) True   Levodopa (unlike dopamine) can enter nerve terminals in
    b) False   the basal ganglia where it undergoes decarboxylation to
    c) False   form dopamine
    d) True   – Entacapone is a catechol-*O*-methyltransferase inhibitor
    e) True

111 a) True   The dose of levodopa is titrated upwards, balancing
    b) True   efficacy against adverse effects. Nausea and vomiting are
    c) False   reduced by the addition of a dopa decarboxylase inhibitor
    d) False   and taking the drug after food
    e) True

112 a) False   Bromocriptine may be used as an initial treatment in
    b) True   Parkinson's disease, particularly in younger patients
    c) False   (<70 years) or as an adjunct with levodopa–dopa
    d) False   decarboxylase combinations in patients with severe motor
    e) True   fluctuations. There is great inter-individual variation in its efficacy. Ropinirole is another dopamine D_2 receptor agonist

113 **a)** True   Selegiline, an MAO-B inhibitor, may slow disease
      b) False   progression in idiopathic Parkinson's disease. It usually
      c) False   allows dose reduction and prolongs the duration of action of
      d) False   levodopa. Oral selegiline is well absorbed (100 per cent) and
      e) False   extensively metabolized in the liver. Rarely hypertension has
been reported. Amantadine (which stimulates release of
endogenous dopamine) potentiates its anti-Parkinson effects

114 **a)** False   Donepezil is used for Alzheimer's disease. Riluzole is used
      b) False   in motor neuron disease. Treatment of spasticity is seldom
      c) True   very effective, but physiotherapy or limited surgical release
      d) True   procedures have some place. The drugs used to reduce
      e) True   spasticity have considerable limitations. Diazepam is
sedative, baclofen is less sedative at equi-effective doses
but can cause vertigo, nausea and hypotension. Intrathecal
baclofen is currently being evaluated. Dantrolene is less
useful for spasticity as it markedly reduces muscle power.
It is used in the management of neuroleptic malignant
syndrome and malignant hyperthermia

115 **a)** True   Tardive dyskinesia is thought to result from the
      b) True   development of 'denervation hypersensitivity' in
      c) True   dopaminergic postsynaptic receptors of the nigrostriatal
      d) False   pathway following chronic receptor blockade by
      e) False   neuroleptics. It is therefore due to a relative preponderance of
dopaminergic effects. Botulinum toxin A is one of the
neurotoxins produced by *Clostridium botulinum* and is used to
treat blepharospasm, certain other dystonias and dynamic
equinus foot deformities due to spasticity in ambulant
paediatric cerebral palsy patients. It blocks the release of
acetylcholine at the neuromuscular junction and is given by
local intramuscular injection. This is a specialist field!

116 **a)** True   Myasthenia gravis is a syndrome of increased muscle
      b) True   fatigability and weakness of striated muscle and results
      c) True   from an autoimmune process with antibodies to nicotinic
      d) False   acetylcholine receptors
      e) True

117 **a)** True   Clinically the distinction between a deficiency (myasthenic
      b) True   crisis) or an excess (cholinergic crisis) may be difficult and
      c) True   improvement with an injection of the very short-acting
      d) True   anticholinesterase edrophonium is diagnostic of
      e) False   myasthenic crisis. Because of its short duration of action,
any deterioration of a cholinergic crisis is unlikely to have
serious consequences although facilities for artificial
ventilation must be available. NB: cholinesterase inhibitors
cause pupillary constriction

118 a) True   Acetylcholinesterase-inhibiting drugs can slow down the
     b) True   progression of mild and moderate Alzheimer's disease, but
     c) True   the benefit is small and only temporary. Memantine, an
     d) False   NMDA receptor antagonist, inhibits glutamate transmission
     e) True   and is licensed for moderate to severe dementia in
                   Alzheimer's disease

119 a) True   See Table 2 for choice of drug in various forms of seizure.
     b) True   Topiramate has been associated with acute myopia with
     c) True   secondary angle-closure glaucoma
     d) True
     e) False

Table 2 Choice of drug in various forms of seizure

Form of seizure	First line	Second line
Partial seizures ± secondary generalized tonic clonic seizures	Valproate Carbamazepine Lamotrigine	Phenytoin Topiramate Tiagabine
Generalized seizures		
Primary (tonic clonic)	Valproate Lamotrigine	Carbamazepine Topiramate Phenytoin
Absence seizures	Ethosuximide Valproate	Lamotrigine Clobazam / Clonazepam
Myoclonic jerks	Valproate	Lamotrigine Clobazam / Clonazepam

Note: Other antiepileptics not listed above may be useful. Refer to National Institute for Health and Clinical Excellence (NICE) guidelines.

120 a) True   Tremor, ataxia and incoordination are dose related. The
     b) True   gastrointestinal effects can be reduced by the use of an
     c) False   enteric coated formulation
     d) False
     e) True

121 a) True   High blood concentrations of phenytoin produce a
     b) True   cerebellar syndrome, involuntary movements and sedation.
     c) True   Macrocytic anaemia which responds to folate is common.
     d) False   Rashes, fever, hepatitis, gum hypertrophy, hirsutism and
     e) True   lymphadenopathy are all well-recognized adverse effects
                   of phenytoin

122 a) True   Age, body weight, sex and, in particular, saturable
     b) False   metabolism which is under polygenic control, contribute to
     c) False   the wide variation in handling of phenytoin
     d) False
     e) True

123 a) False
b) False
c) True
d) False
e) True

In addition to its effectiveness in many forms of epilepsy except absence seizures, carbamazepine is effective in trigeminal neuralgia. It induces its own metabolism, hence the half-life after a single dose is 25–60 hours, but on chronic dosing this falls to 10 hours

124 a) False
b) True
c) True
d) True
e) True

Carbamazepine commonly causes adverse effects but these are seldom severe. They are particularly troublesome early in treatment and may resolve without alteration of dose which is probably related to the induction of its own metabolism, although pharmacodynamic tolerance is also a factor. Carbamazepine therapy should be initiated at a low dose and titrated upwards slowly depending on response. Hyponatraemia is caused by stimulation of antidiuretic hormone secretion

125 a) False
b) True
c) False
d) True
e) False

Sodium valproate is effective against several forms of epilepsy. Adverse effects most commonly involve the alimentary system. These include nausea, vomiting and abdominal pain (which may be reduced by enteric coated tablets). Use in pregnancy is associated with increased neural tube defects. To reduce the risk of neural tube defects, folate supplements are advised before and during pregnancy in women on antiepileptic drugs

126 a) True
b) True
c) True
d) True
e) False

Vigabatrin is reserved for the treatment of epilepsy unsatisfactorily controlled by more established drugs. It is associated with visual field defects. Onset of symptoms varies from one month to several years after starting treatment. Unlike most anticonvulsants it is not metabolized by the liver and is excreted unchanged by the kidney

127 a) True
b) True
c) False
d) True
e) False

Women on long-term enzyme-inducing drugs who are unable to use an alternative reliable method of contraception should use an oral contraceptive containing at least 50 μg ethinylestradiol under expert family planning supervision. Enzyme induction is also the basis of anticonvulsant osteomalacia (extremely rare) due to reduced serum 25-hydroxycholecalciferol

128 a) True
b) False
c) True
d) False
e) False

Status epilepticus is a medical emergency with a mortality of about 10 per cent. Rapid suppression of seizure activity can usually be achieved with intravenous lorazepam. False teeth should be removed, an airway established and oxygen (60 per cent) administered as soon as possible

129 a) True
b) True

Uncomplicated febrile seizures have an excellent prognosis. It is usual to reduce fever using paracetamol,

c) False removal of clothing, tepid sponging and fanning
d) False
e) False

130 a) True Oral aspirin, NSAID or paracetamol is effective in the
b) False treatment of the headache of acute migraine in nearly
c) True 75 per cent of patients. During a migraine attack, gastric statis
d) True occurs, hence the popularity of a combination of aspirin or
e) False paracetamol with metoclopramide (a dopamine antagonist)
which enhances gastric emptying as well as counteracting
the nausea common in migraine. The value of ergotamine
is very limited. There is a risk of peripheral vasospasm

131 a) True Sumatriptan is a selective agonist of $5HT_{1D}$ receptors,
b) True which are found predominantly in the cranial circulation.
c) True Prepacked dosage vials are available for subcutaneous
d) True self-injection. Sumatriptan is only 14 per cent available
e) False after oral administration. A nasal spray is also available.
The half-life is 2 hours. Headache recurs after a single dose
in 30–40 per cent of patients

132 a) False Pizotifen is given at night as its principal adverse effect
b) False is drowsiness. It also increases appetite and causes
c) True weight gain. Beta blockers potentiate the peripheral
d) True vasoconstriction caused by ergotamine and these drugs
e) True should not be given concurrently. Ergotamine must not be
used for prophylaxis. Methysergide has $5HT_2$ antagonist
activity with partial 5HT agonist activity. It should only be
used under specialist hospital supervision. Retroperitoneal
fibrosis may lead to renal failure

133 a) True Halothane is a potent anaesthetic but weak analgesic. It has
b) False a low therapeutic index. In many centres in the UK
c) True sevoflurane is the inhalation anaesthetic of first choice
d) False
e) True

134 a) True Fentanyl is a synthetic opioid and is commonly used as an
b) False analgesic supplement. Its short duration of action (peak
c) True effect 20–30 minutes) is explained by redistribution from
d) False the brain. The half-life is 2–4 hours. It undergoes hepatic
e) True metabolism

135 a) False Nitrous oxide is commonly combined with volatile
b) True anaesthetics for its analgesic properties. Premixed nitrous
c) True oxide and oxygen mixtures are used in obstetric practice
d) False and by ambulance drivers
e) False

136 a) False
b) False
c) True
d) True
e) True

Thiopental sodium, an ultra short-acting barbiturate, is used primarily as an induction agent. Propofol is used for induction, maintenance of anaesthesia and sedation in intensive care units

137 a) True
b) True
c) True
d) False
e) False

The chief aim of premedication is to allay anxiety in the patient awaiting surgery. Inadequate premedication may lead to the administration of larger doses of anaesthetic than would otherwise have been required, resulting in delayed recovery. Neostigmine, an anticholinesterase, may be used at the end of a procedure to reverse non-depolarizing muscle relaxants such as tubocurarine. Ketamine is a parenteral anaesthetic which has a wide therapeutic index. Although it is a potent analgesic and sedative it can cause vivid unpleasant hallucinations which may recur for months. It increases muscle tone and blood pressure. It is useful in major disasters for rapid, safe anaesthesia of trapped casualties to carry out procedures such as amputation

138 a) True
b) False
c) True
d) False
e) False

Atracurium has a rapid onset of action. It occasionally causes histamine release leading to flushing of the face and chest, hypotension and rarely bronchospasm. Continuous infusion is popular in intensive care. It is inactivated spontaneously in the plasma, which is a valuable property in hepatic and renal failure

139 a) False
b) True
c) False
d) True
e) False

Opioids may cause fatal respiratory depression. Even epidural opioids can cause respiratory depression and in this situation epidural 'local' anaesthesia and intramuscular NSAIDs are preferred

140 a) True
b) True
c) True
d) True
e) True

Malignant hyperthermia is a rare but potentially lethal complication of anaesthesia. It consists of a rapid increase in body temperature accompanied by tachycardia and generalized muscle spasm. Severe acidosis and hyperkalaemia occur. Dantrolene reverses the muscle spasm

141 a) True
b) False
c) False
d) False
e) True

Small unmyelinated fibres are depressed first, hence the order of loss of function is pain, temperature, touch, proprioception and motor function. Lidocaine does not affect vascular smooth muscle but is available with adrenaline, a vasoconstrictor which prolongs its local effect. This combination may cause vasospasm and severe digital ischaemia if used for a 'ring' block, hence the combination is contraindicated in this situation. Bupivacaine is a long-acting local anaesthetic which is often used for peripheral nerve, plexus, epidural and spinal anaesthesia. Toxicity includes cardiac dysrhythmias

142
a) True
b) False
c) True
d) True
e) True

Paracetamol probably produces its analgesic effect by central inhibition of cyclo-oxygenase. It is antipyretic but not anti-inflammatory

143
a) True
b) True
c) False
d) True
e) True

Gastric irritation is reduced by taking aspirin after food

144
a) False
b) True
c) False
d) True
e) True

The commonest adverse effect associated with salicylates is dyspepsia. Chronic blood loss from the stomach may be asymptomatic. Salicylism which is associated with high blood concentrations, consists of tinnitus, deafness, nausea, vomiting and occasionally abdominal pain and flushing

145
a) True
b) True
c) True
d) True
e) True

Ibuprofen is an NSAID which is available without prescription. The side-effects are those of all the NSAIDs, of which gastrointestinal irritation is the most common. Selective inhibitors of cyclo-oxygenase 2 (COX 2), e.g. celecoxib, may improve gastrointestinal tolerance, but are associated with an increased incidence of cardiovascular events

146
a) False
b) False
c) False
d) True
e) True

Nefopam is chemically and pharmacologically unrelated to opioids and NSAIDs. It is used for moderately severe pain. It can cause fatal hypertension if prescribed during or within two weeks of cessation of non-selective MAO inhibitor treatment

147
a) False
b) True
c) False
d) False
e) False

Co-codamol, a compound analgesic of codeine phosphate and paracetamol, is widely prescribed. If the codeine content/tablet is 8 mg it is available without prescription. When taking a drug history one must be aware that many over-the-counter remedies contain a surprising mixture of pharmacologically active agents, although sometimes in almost 'homeopathic' quantities

148
a) True
b) True
c) False
d) True
e) True

The most important use of morphine is pain relief. It is of particular value in palliative care. The use of oral modified-release preparations allows twice-daily dosing whereas if the standard solution is used it needs to be given every 4 hours

149
a) True
b) True

Patients with decreased respiratory reserve and myxoedema are also more sensitive

c) True
d) True
e) False

150 a) False
     b) True
     c) True
     d) True
     e) False

Morphine increases smooth muscle tone throughout the gastrointestinal tract and in addition reduces peristalsis through an action on the receptors in the ganglion plexus in the gut wall which results in constipation. Diamorphine is diacetylmorphine. Its actions are similar to those of morphine but is more potent as an analgesic when given by injection. It is more soluble than morphine. Diamorphine and 6-acetylmorphine enter the brain more rapidly than morphine

151 a) False
     b) False
     c) False
     d) False
     e) False

Pethidine causes similar respiratory depression and vomiting to morphine, but does not release histamine or suppress cough and only uncommonly produces pupillary constriction to the same extent as morphine

152 a) False
     b) False
     c) True
     d) True
     e) True

Morphine is a metabolite of codeine. Codeine is used as an analgesic, cough suppressant and antidiarrhoeal agent. The plasma half-life is 3–4 hours. It is metabolized by CYP2D6. It is less effective in patients deficient in CYP2D6

153 a) True
     b) True
     c) False
     d) True
     e) True

In common with other partial agonists buprenorphine occupies a much larger fraction of the receptors to produce its analgesic effect than does a full agonist. Consequently it can precipitate pain and cause withdrawal symptoms in patients who have received other opioids and relatively much larger doses of naloxone are required to displace it from receptors in overdosage compared to a full agonist

154 a) True
     b) False
     c) True
     d) False
     e) False

Naloxone is a pure competitive antagonist. It has a half-life of 1 hour which is less than many opioids

EMQ ANSWERS

155 CENTRALLY ACTIVE DRUGS

1 G Sumatriptan is a $5HT_1$ antagonist. Sumatriptan can be given by mouth, subcutaneous injection or as a nasal spray during a migraine attack. Sumatriptan and other $5HT_1$ agonists (rizatriptan and zolmitriptan) can cause vasoconstriction in coronary and pulmonary vascular beds.

2 J Valproate is the first-choice anticonvulsant for myoclonic jerks. It is effective against many forms of epilepsy.

3 H Tardive dyskinesias follow months or years of conventional (D_2 blocking) antipsychotic treatment. Anticholinergics aggravate symptoms. The D_2 blocker should be stopped, but structural changes (possible increased sensitivity of presynaptic dopamine receptors) occur and may be irreversible. An atypical antipsychotic (e.g. aripiprazole) may help alleviate the symptoms and should help maintain control of the schizophrenia.

4 C An SSRI such as citalopram is usually effective in depression and much safer in overdose than a tricyclic antidepressant (e.g. imipramine).

5 A A short-acting benzodiazepine such as temazepam is the treatment of choice for severe disabling insomnia.

156 DRUG-INDUCED MOVEMENT DISORDERS

1 C Salbutamol, a $beta_2$ agonist, commonly causes a dose-related tremor. Other drug causes include caffeine, thyroxine, SSRIs (e.g. fluoxetine), valproate, lithium and withdrawal from alcohol and benzodiazepines.

2 I Phenytoin, an antiepileptic, causes dose-related ataxia with cerebellar signs including nystagmus (as does alcohol intoxication).

3 E Aminoglycosides, e.g. gentamicin, cause 8th nerve damage, which can affect hearing and balance. 8th nerve toxicity correlates with trough drug blood levels.

4 G The commonest drug causes of proximal myopathy are chronic corticosteroid therapy and alcoholism.

5 B Tendon damage including rupture has been associated with fluoroquinolone (e.g. ciprofloxacin) therapy. Elderly patients and those on concurrent corticosteroids are most at risk.

157 TREATMENT OF MOVEMENT DISORDERS AND DEMENTIA

1 G Ropinirole is a dopamine receptor agonist which is often used as initial treatment in younger (<70 years) patients with parkinsonism.

2 A Botulinum toxin (A and B) is a neurotoxin. It irreversibly blocks the release of acetylcholine at the neuromuscular junction. It is often used in cosmetic clinics.

3 J Neostigmine and pyridostigmine are cholinesterase inhibitors.

4 B Procyclidine is an antimuscarinic of value in treating antipsychotic drug-induced acute dystonias.

5 C Donepezil has a limited effect on slowing the speed of progression of Alzheimer's disease.

158 ANALGESICS/PAIN

1 H Paracetamol is a mild analgesic and antipyretic which, unlike aspirin, is not associated with Reye's syndrome. Therapeutic doses are extremely well tolerated but overdose can be fatal usually through hepatic failure.

2 F Indometacin, an NSAID, is effective in acute gout.

3 G Patient-controlled analgesia using morphine is especially valuable in the management of post-operative visceral pain.

4 B Aspirin overdose is associated with tinnitus.

5 A Fentanyl, a potent synthetic opioid, is available as a transdermal patch which can provide analgesia for up to 72 hours.

CHAPTER THREE

MUSCULOSKELETAL SYSTEM

MULTIPLE CHOICE QUESTIONS

159 Gold salts when used in the treatment of progressive rheumatoid arthritis:

a) Are usually administered daily by intravenous injection
b) If effective, benefit should be observed after the first week of treatment
c) Produce objective improvement in about 75 per cent of patients
d) Can cause skin rashes which can necessitate treatment cessation
e) If they cause stomatitis this may be due to neutropenia

160 Penicillamine is used in the management of:

a) Rheumatoid arthritis
b) Systemic lupus erythematosus (SLE)
c) Wilson's disease
d) Cystinuria
e) Lead poisoning

161 Adverse effects associated with penicillamine include:

a) Thrombocytopenia
b) Leucopenia
c) Immune complex glomerulonephritis
d) Loss of taste
e) Myasthenia gravis

162 Etanercept:

a) Is a humanized monoclonal antibody against tumour necrosis factor alpha (TNF-α)
b) Can cause life-threatening hypersensitivity reactions
c) Has a half-life of 5–13 days
d) Can cause pancytopenia
e) Is rarely associated with a demyelinating syndrome

163 The following are likely to be effective in the treatment of an acute episode of gout:
a) Indometacin
b) Naproxen
c) Alendronate
d) Probenecid
e) Colchicine

164 The following may cause hyperuricaemia:
a) Sulfinpyrazone
b) Cytosine arabinoside when treating acute leukaemia
c) Bendromethiazide
d) Low-dose aspirin
e) Bezafibrate

165 Allopurinol:
a) Inhibits xanthine oxidase
b) May precipitate acute gout
c) Is contraindicated in renal failure
d) Should not be prescribed with a non-steroidal anti-inflammatory drug (NSAID)
e) Blocks the metabolic inactivation of suxamethonium

166 In a patient with osteoarthritis:
a) Physical exercise and weight loss can be helpful
b) NSAIDs are contraindicated
c) Gold therapy reverses the pathophysiology of the disease
d) Symptoms are exacerbated by bisphosphonates, e.g. alendronate
e) Raloxifene may slow disease progression

167 Indometacin causes the following adverse effects:
a) Biochemical hepatitis
b) Spuriously increased serum creatinine
c) Hypokalaemia
d) Exacerbates cardiac failure
e) Antagonizes the antihypertensive effects of angiotensin-converting enzyme (ACE) inhibitors

Answers: see pages 72–73

EXTENDED MATCHING QUESTIONS

168 ARTHRITIS

A	Colchicine	**F**	Methylprednisolone
B	Azathioprine	**G**	Hydroxychloroquine
C	Allopurinol	**H**	Naproxen
D	Gold injections	**I**	D-penicillamine
E	Methotrexate	**J**	Etanercept

Link each of 1 to 5 below with the most appropriate item from A to J:

1 Chronic use can cause cirrhosis
2 Used before commencing chemotherapy of leukaemia
3 Licensed for severe ankylosing spondylitis inadequately responsive to conventional therapy
4 Intra-articular injection in rheumatoid arthritis
5 Used in familial Mediterranean fever

ANSWERS: see pages 73–74

ANSWERS

MCQ ANSWERS

159 a) False   Gold (as sodium aurothiomalate) is usually administered
     b) False   as weekly intramuscular injections or by mouth daily.
     c) True   Benefit is not anticipated for at least six weeks. Blood
     d) True   dyscrasias and glomerular injury (nephrotic syndrome)
     e) True   occur and monitoring of blood counts and urine is
                performed monthly. Rashes may progress to
                exfoliation

160 a) True   Penicillamine, a breakdown product of penicillin, is given
     b) False   by mouth. In rheumatoid arthritis clinical improvement is
     c) True   anticipated only after 6–12 weeks. It is contraindicated in
     d) True   SLE. Apart from its immunosuppressive action, it also
     e) True   chelates certain heavy metals (Cu, Pb, etc.)

161 a) True   The toxicity of penicillamine is such that it should only be
     b) True   used by clinicians with experience of the drug and with
     c) True   meticulous patient monitoring
     d) True
     e) True

162 a) False   – Etanercept is a recombinant protein that has two soluble
                TNF receptors joined to an Fc fragment; this is in contrast
                to infliximab, a humanized murine monoclonal against
                TNF-α used in Crohn's disease. Both are licensed for the
                treatment of adult rheumatoid arthritis
     b) True   – Like all proteins it can cause hypersensitivity reactions
     c) True   – It has a long half-life in plasma and is administered every
                two weeks
     d) True   – It can cause bone marrow suppression (all lineages) and
                sepsis
     e) True   – Rarely, demyelinating syndromes like multiple sclerosis
                have been reported with its use

163 a) True   Acute gout is treated by anti-inflammatory analgesic
     b) True   agents. Colchicine is an alternative in those unable to
     c) False   tolerate NSAIDs but commonly causes diarrhoea.
     d) False   Alendronate is a bisphosphonate used in the
     e) True   management of Paget's disease. Bisphosphonates
                are also used to treat hypercalcaemia of pregnancy. They
                may be used in the prevention of postmenopausal
                osteoporosis

164 a) False   Uric acid is the end product of purine metabolism in humans,
b) True   and gives rise to problems because of its limited solubility.
c) True   Cytosine arabinoside causes massive cell death and increased
d) True   uric acid production. Diuretics, low-dose salicylates and
e) False   pyrazinamide inhibit tubular excretion of uric acid

165 a) True   Allopurinol is used as long-term medication to treat
b) True   patients with recurrent gout. By inhibiting xanthine
c) False   oxidase it decreases uric acid production. It potentiates
d) False   azathioprine by blocking inactivation of its active
e) False   metabolite 6-mercaptopurine

166 a) True
b) False   – NSAIDs are probably one of the most widely used
c) False   treatments although paracetamol, because of its superior
d) False   tolerance in the elderly, should be tried first
e) False   – Raloxifene is used in the treatment and prevention of
postmenopausal osteoporosis

167 a) True   – Can cause transaminitis
b) False   – Reduces glomerular filtration rate (GFR) and truly causes
an increase in serum creatinine by diminishing
vasodilatory prostaglandins in the renal bed
c) False   – Reduces renal potassium excretion thus leads to
hyperkalaemia
d) True   – Reduces Na excretion leading to increased fluid retention
and fluid overload
e) True

EMQ ANSWERS

168 ARTHRITIS

1 E Methotrexate is one of the most frequently used disease-modifying antirheumatic drugs (DMARDs) in rheumatoid arthritis. Myelosuppression is another potentially fatal adverse effect.

2 C As well as being used in the prophylaxis of gout, allopurinol is used before commencing chemotherapy of rapidly dividing malignancies where killing a large number of tumour cells increases nucleic acid breakdown so increasing production of urate which can precipitate in the renal tract. Allopurinol prevents this (xanthine is much more water soluble than urate).

3 J Inhibitors of TNF can reactivate latent tuberculosis as can corticosteroids and other immunosuppressants.

4 F Intra-articular corticosteroids, e.g. methylprednisolone, are valuable to reduce pain, increase mobility and reduce deformity in one or a few joints in a rheumatoid arthritis flare.

5 A Colchicine, in addition to its use in the treatment and prophylaxis of gout, is also effective in the treatment of familial Mediterranean fever.

CHAPTER FOUR

CARDIOVASCULAR SYSTEM

MULTIPLE CHOICE QUESTIONS

169 The following are modifiable risk factors for the genesis of atheromatous plaque:
a) Smoking
b) Obesity
c) Dyslipidaemia
d) Glucose intolerance
e) Hypertension

170 Colestyramine:
a) Causes a fall in plasma cholesterol
b) Increases fecal excretion of bile acids
c) Reduces absorption of folic acid
d) Causes diarrhoea in diabetic autonomic neuropathy
e) Reduces pruritus in incomplete biliary obstruction

171 Bezafibrate:
a) Lowers plasma triglyceride
b) Is ineffective post cholecystectomy
c) Inhibits lipoprotein lipase
d) Is indicated in alcohol-induced hyperlipidaemia
e) Potentiates the effects of warfarin

172 Simvastatin, an HMG-CoA (3-hydroxy-3-methyl-glutaryl-CoA) reductase inhibitor:
a) Lowers low-density lipoprotein (LDL) cholesterol
b) Is particularly useful in heterozygous familial hypercholesterolaemia
c) Acts locally on HMG-CoA reductase in the intestine
d) Is associated with myositis/myopathy
e) Is ineffective if prescribed with ezetimibe

173 The following can cause hypertension:

a) Corticosteroid therapy
b) Oral contraception
c) Alcohol withdrawal
d) Amphetamines
e) Ergotamine

174 Thiazide diuretics when used in the management of uncomplicated essential hypertension:

a) Reduce the risk of stroke
b) Are natriuretic
c) Potassium supplements are usually required
d) Reduce plasma renin
e) Are associated with impotence

175 Beta-adrenoceptor antagonists:

a) Are indicated in patients with stable heart failure
b) Prolong life in survivors of myocardial infarction
c) Improve performance of sprinters
d) The antihypertensive effect is antagonized by non-steroidal anti-inflammatory drugs (NSAIDs)
e) May cause life-threatening bronchospasm in asthmatics

176 The following drugs when used as monotherapy in the management of hypertension are likely to be less effective in Afro-Caribbean than in white patients:

a) Atenolol
b) Enalapril
c) Bendroflumethiazide
d) Amlodipine
e) Diltiazem

177 Ramipril, an angiotensin-converting enzyme (ACE) inhibitor:

a) Reduces concentrations of angiotensin II
b) Increases concentrations of bradykinin
c) Increases noradrenaline release from sympathetic nerve terminals
d) Increases aldosterone secretion
e) Causes hypokalaemia

178 Irbesartan (an angiotensin-11 receptor antagonist) is contraindicated in:

a) Left ventricular failure
b) Asthma
c) Bilateral renal artery stenosis
d) Pregnancy
e) Diabetic nephropathy

179 Nifedipine, a dihydropyridine calcium channel blocker:
- **a)** Dilates veins more than arteries
- **b)** Can be combined with beta blockers in the management of hypertension
- **c)** Increases plasma calcium concentration
- **d)** Is contraindicated in asthma
- **e)** Raises the plasma concentration of cholesterol

180 Nifedipine in comparison to verapamil is more likely to:
- **a)** Worsen angina
- **b)** Cause ankle swelling unresponsive to diuretics
- **c)** Have negative inotropic effects
- **d)** Cause flushing and headache
- **e)** Cause constipation

181 Doxazosin:
- **a)** Is a selective reversible α_1 receptor antagonist
- **b)** Should always be prescribed with a beta blocker to prevent reflex tachycardia
- **c)** Is associated with first-dose hypotension
- **d)** Reduces plasma LDL/high-density lipoprotein (HDL) cholesterol ratio
- **e)** Can cause urinary incontinence in women with pre-existing pelvic pathology

182 Sodium nitroprusside:
- **a)** Is administered by intravenous infusion
- **b)** Prolonged administration can lead to cyanide poisoning
- **c)** Has a half-life of about one week
- **d)** Reduces cardiac 'pre-load'
- **e)** Reduces cardiac 'afterload'

183 Methyldopa:
- **a)** Causes central α_2 agonist effects
- **b)** Causes drowsiness and fatigue
- **c)** Pyrexia is an adverse effect
- **d)** Is associated with Coombs'-positive haemolytic anaemia
- **e)** A single missed dose can cause profound rebound hypertension

184 The following hypotensive combinations are rational when a single drug has not been effective in treating essential hypertension:
- **a)** Thiazide and candesartan
- **b)** Thiazide and ramipril in an asthmatic
- **c)** Amiloride and ramipril in an asthmatic who has gout
- **d)** Nifedipine and verapamil in a man who has had thiazide-induced impotence, second-degree heart block and captopril-induced rash
- **e)** Ramipril and doxazosin in a man with prostatism

185 The following drug effects have been correctly paired with the named drug:

a) Hydralazine – drug-induced systemic lupus erythematosus (SLE)
b) Minoxidil – hirsutism
c) Captopril – first-dose hypotension
d) Atenolol – tremor
e) Candesartan – cough

186 Management of acute ST elevation myocardial infarction (STEMI) should usually include:

a) 24 per cent oxygen
b) Intravenous opiate with an antiemetic
c) Aspirin
d) Some measure to open the coronary atery (e.g. angioplasty)
e) Lidocaine (lignocaine)

187 The management of unstable angina usually includes:

a) Aspirin
b) Glyceryl trinitrate (GTN)
c) Low molecular weight heparin
d) Salbutamol
e) Beta-adrenoceptor antagonist

188 GTN:

a) Relaxes vascular smooth muscle
b) Is associated with tolerance more commonly with transdermal GTN patches than sublingual GTN
c) Is volatile
d) Is more selective for arteriolar than for venous smooth muscle
e) May relieve the pain of oesophageal spasm

189 Beta-adrenoceptor antagonists:

a) Increase cardiac tissue cyclic adenosine monophosphate (cAMP)
b) Competitively antagonize the β receptor-mediated effects of adrenaline and noradrenaline
c) Non-competitively antagonize several of the actions of thyroxine
d) Decrease peripheral vascular resistance
e) Reduce renin secretion

190 The following drugs may reduce the risk of recurrence or death post myocardial infarction:

a) Aspirin
b) Beta blockers
c) Dexfenfluramine
d) Sildenafil
e) Statins

191 Verapamil is used:
  a) For prophylaxis of angina
  b) To treat hypertension
  c) To treat ventricular tachycardia
  d) To prevent cerebral vasospasm following subarachnoid haemorrhage
  e) To treat left ventricular failure

192 A calcium channel blocker such as amlodipine or nifedipine is preferred to a beta blocker such as atenolol to treat hypertension and angina in patients who also have:
  a) Chronic bronchitis
  b) Peripheral vascular disease
  c) Heart block
  d) Diabetes
  e) Anxiety

193 Aspirin:
  a) Reduces the risk of stroke in patients with transient ischaemic attacks
  b) Predisposes to peptic ulceration
  c) Irreversibly inhibits fatty acid cyclo-oxygenase
  d) Has no effect on bleeding time
  e) Needs to be given twice daily to prevent platelet cyclo-oxygenase resynthesis within the dose interval

194 Streptokinase:
  a) Is derived from streptococci
  b) Reduces the acute mortality of myocardial infarction only if administered within 4 hours of the onset of chest pain
  c) Is contraindicated if the patient is taking regular NSAID therapy
  d) Is administered by intravenous infusion
  e) Should not be given to patients over the age of 60 years

195 Alteplase:
  a) Is a prodrug that liberates streptokinase
  b) Heparin must not be administered within 24 hours of alteplase infusion
  c) Should only be administered if pulmonary artery pressure can be measured
  d) Is indicated in the treatment of pulmonary embolism
  e) Is contraindicated if aspirin has been administered in the last 24 hours

196 The following are relative contraindications to the use of streptokinase in acute myocardial infarction:

a) Therapy with streptokinase from 5 days to 12 months previously
b) Stroke due to cerebral thrombosis in the last six months
c) Concurrent hormone replacement therapy for menopausal symptoms
d) Pulmonary disease with cavitation
e) Penicillin allergy

197 Unfractionated heparin:

a) Binds to antithrombin III
b) Inhibits the action of thrombin
c) Is monitored in the laboratory by measurement of activated partial thromboplastin time (APTT)
d) Is less effective in patients with inherited or acquired deficiency of antithrombin III
e) Is reversed by protamine sulphate

198 Low molecular weight heparin (LMWH) prophylaxis to prevent deep vein thrombosis/pulmonary embolism in major surgery:

a) Must be started one week before surgery
b) Is via twice-daily intramuscular injection
c) Is more likely to be of value in an obese man of 50 than in a slim man of 30
d) Unfractionated heparin should be substituted for LMWH in renal failure
e) Concomitant antibiotics are contraindicated

199 The following are recognized adverse effects of unfractionated heparin therapy:

a) Osteoporosis
b) Alopecia
c) Thrombocytopenia
d) Diarrhoea
e) Fetal cleft palate

200 The following statements are correct:

a) Thrombocytopenia is more commonly associated with unfractionated heparin than LMWH
b) LMWH is eliminated solely by renal excretion
c) Neither heparin nor LMWH cross the placenta
d) Fondaparinux selectively binds and inhibits factor Xa
e) Hirudin is a direct thrombin inhibitor

201 Warfarin:

a) Prevents the hepatic synthesis of the vitamin K-dependent coagulation factors II, VII, IX and X
b) Is structurally closely related to vitamin K
c) Should initially be given as a subcutaneous loading dose
d) During life-threatening bleeding can be reversed by vitamin K and fresh frozen plasma
e) Anticoagulant effect is monitored by measurement of the prothrombin time/international normalized ratio (INR)

202 The following are relative or absolute contraindications to warfarin therapy:

a) First trimester of pregnancy
b) Prosthetic heart valves
c) Space-occupying CNS lesion
d) Concurrent digoxin therapy
e) Glucose 6-phosphate dehydrogenase (G6PD) deficiency

203 The following inhibit the metabolism of warfarin:

a) Cimetidine
b) Fluvoxamine
c) St John's wort
d) Carbamazepine
e) Smoking

204 The following inhibit platelet activation and/or aggregation:

a) Warfarin
b) Heparin
c) Thromboxane A_2
d) Prostacyclin (epoprostenol)
e) Dipyridamole

205 Clopidogrel:

a) Is a direct inhibitor of glycoprotein IIb and IIIa
b) The antiplatelet effect lasts the life of the platelet
c) Is usually given by intravenous bolus in acute coronary syndrome
d) Is a prodrug, requiring conversion in the liver to its active metabolite
e) Prolongs the QTc (QT interval on the ECG corrected for heart rate) predisposing to ventricular tachycardia

206 Prostacyclin (epoprostenol):

a) Relaxes pulmonary and systemic vasculature
b) Is the principal endogenous prostaglandin of large- and medium-sized blood vessels
c) Is an effective anticoagulant
d) Is contraindicated in haemodialysis
e) Increases diastolic pressure

207 The principal beneficial effect in heart failure of the following drugs is to reduce preload (left ventricular filling pressure):

a) Digoxin
b) Furosemide
c) Dobutamine
d) GTN
e) Sodium nitroprusside

208 The following drugs at standard therapeutic doses aggravate heart failure:

a) Imatinib (a tyrosine kinase inhibitor)
b) Verapamil
c) Daunorubicin
d) Ibuprofen
e) Bendroflumethiazide

209 In acute pulmonary oedema the following are usually appropriate:

a) Sublingual nifedipine
b) Lie the patient supine
c) Oxygen
d) Intravenous loop diuretic
e) Intravenous morphine

210 Intravenous furosemide:

a) Causes natriuresis
b) Causes kaliuresis
c) Has an indirect vasodilator effect
d) Diuresis begins 10–20 minutes after an intravenous dose
e) High doses are ototoxic

211 ACE inhibitors:

a) Are positive inotropes
b) Increase afterload
c) Increase preload
d) May cause cough
e) Should be given parenterally in acute heart failure

212 The following statements concerning drugs in heart failure are correct:

a) The combination of furosemide (a loop diuretic) and ramipril (an ACE inhibitor) should be avoided
b) Candesartan (an angiotensin-II receptor antagonist) is generally better tolerated than captopril (an ACE inhibitor)
c) Beta blockers are contraindicated in heart failure
d) The combination of loop diuretic, ACE inhibitor and spironolactone must always be avoided because of the risk of hyperkalaemia
e) The combination of hydralazine and nitrates is of demonstrated efficacy in African-origin patients

213 Dobutamine:

a) Is a sympathomimetic amine
b) Is predominantly a β_1-receptor agonist
c) Increases blood pressure via vasoconstriction
d) Should not be given at the same time as loop diuretics
e) Increases myocardial oxygen consumption

214 The following drugs can cause sinus tachycardia:

a) Esmolol
b) Theophylline
c) Ephedrine
d) Amphetamine
e) Verapamil

215 Lidocaine:

a) Is a class 1b agent that blocks cardiac Na^+ channels, reducing the rate of rise of the cardiac action potential and increasing the effective refractory period
b) Is epileptogenic
c) Is a positive inotrope
d) Is usually administered as an intravenous bolus followed by infusion
e) Is the drug of first choice for supraventricular tachycardia

216 The following drugs prolong the QT interval and/or cause torsades de pointes:

a) Erythromycin
b) Pimozide
c) Foscarnet
d) Tacrolimus
e) Disopyramide

217 Amiodarone:

a) Is effective in resistant atrial fibrillation or flutter
b) Is effective in preventing recurrent ventricular fibrillation
c) Is contraindicated in Wolff–Parkinson–White (WPW) syndrome
d) May be given intravenously via a central line
e) Prolongs the QT interval

218 The following adverse effects are associated with amiodarone:

a) Visual disturbances (e.g. coloured halos)
b) Hyperthyroidism
c) Hypothyroidism
d) Pulmonary fibrosis
e) Photosensitivity

219 Amiodarone:

  a) Is highly lipid soluble

  b) Has an apparent volume of distribution of approximately 5000 L

  c) Is predominantly eliminated by the kidney

  d) Accumulates in the heart

  e) Has a half-life of 3 weeks

220 Sotalol:

  a) Is effective in supraventricular and ventricular dysrhythmias

  b) Is not effective when given by mouth

  c) The dose should be reduced in renal impairment

  d) May cause torsade de pointes

  e) Is a less potent negative inotrope than amiodarone

221 Intravenous verapamil:

  a) May terminate supraventricular tachycardia

  b) Must not be given to patients receiving beta blockers

  c) Reduces digoxin excretion

  d) One must delay DC cardioversion at least 2 hours after a dose

  e) Shortens the PR interval on the ECG

222 Adenosine:

  a) Is used to terminate ventricular tachycardia

  b) Is contraindicated in regular broad complex tachycardia

  c) Dilates bronchial smooth muscle

  d) Is associated with chest pain

  e) Circulatory effects last 20–30 seconds

223 Digoxin:

  a) Reduces the ventricular rate in atrial fibrillation

  b) Is contraindicated in second-degree heart block

  c) Is the treatment of choice in atrial fibrillation in a patient with WPW syndrome

  d) Induced dysrhythmias may be terminated by magnesium

  e) 80 per cent of administered digoxin is excreted unchanged in the bile

224 A 70-year-old woman has recurrent, symptomatic ventricular tachycardia following an acute myocardial infarction in spite of DC conversion and lidocaine. The following may be effective:

  a) Amiodarone

  b) Atropine

  c) Verapamil

  d) Adenosine

  e) Isoprenaline

225 The following are indications for transvenous pacing:
   a) Asymptomatic sinus bradycardia post inferior myocardial infarction
   b) First-degree heart block post inferior myocardial infarction
   c) A heart rate of 34 bpm at rest in an athlete with second-degree (Mobitz type 1) heart block
   d) Asymptomatic congenital complete heart block
   e) Blackouts associated with bradycardia in sick sinus syndrome

226 The following dysrhythmias are correctly paired with their first-line treatment:
   a) Ventricular fibrillation – synchronized DC cardioversion
   b) Ventricular fibrillation – unsynchronized DC cardioversion
   c) Ventricular tachycardia post myocardial infarction – esmolol
   d) Rapid chronic (established) atrial fibrillation – flecainide
   e) Drug-induced torsade de pointes – disopyramide

Answers: see pages 89–97

EXTENDED MATCHING QUESTIONS

227 ATHEROMA AND THROMBOSIS

A Simvastatin
B Recombinant hirudin
C Tranexamic acid
D Epoprostenol (prostacyclin)
E Estradiol

F Fenofibrate
G Warfarin
H Colestyramine
I Tissue plasminogen activator
J Ezetimibe

Link each of 1 to 5 below with the most appropriate item from A to J:

1 Useful combined with a statin
2 Inhibition of platelet aggregation during haemodialysis
3 Lowers serum triglyceride and cholesterol concentrations
4 Causes malabsorption of fat-soluble vitamins
5 Myalgia

228 HYPERTENSION

A Labetalol
B Minoxidil
C Doxazosin
D Methyldopa
E Atenolol

F Spironolactone
G Candesartan
H Trandolapril
I Bendroflumethiazide
J Amlodipine

Select the drug from the list above most appropriate to prescribe to the patients described below. In each patient the current blood pressure is above 'target'.

1 A 40-year-old Afro-Caribbean man who has poorly controlled hypertension having stopped bendroflumethiazide, which caused impotence
2 A 70-year-old white man who takes losartan and amlodipine and who has symptoms from prostatic hyperplasia
3 A 50-year-old hypertensive man who has hyperaldosteronism due to bilateral adrenal hyperplasia who is currently on no therapy
4 A 50-year-old white man who has type II diabetes and asthma. He currently takes gliclazide, simvastatin and inhaled beclomethasone. He was on trandolapril, but this was associated with a troublesome cough
5 A 50-year-old Afro-Caribbean woman who developed marked lower limb oedema on amlodipine

229 ISCHAEMIC HEART DISEASE

A	Ramipril	F	Nifedipine
B	Warfarin	G	Verapamil
C	Tissue plasminogen activator	H	Nicorandil
D	Glyceryl trinitrate	I	Simvastatin
E	Magnesium	J	None of the above

Which of the above drugs is useful in each of the following clinical situations?

1 Acute treatment of an angina attack in a 65-year-old man with ischaemic chest pain following exertion

2 Acute treatment of anterior ST-elevation myocardial infarction in a previously healthy 60-year-old man

3 Long-term treatment of left ventricular dysfunction in a 65-year-old woman post myocardial infarction

4 Long-term prevention of cardiac events in an asymptomatic 67-year-old woman with a 10-year history of type 2 diabetes and a total cholesterol of 5.0 mmol/L

5 Prevention of angina in a 78-year-old man with widespread diffuse coronary artery disease, not amenable to percutaneous coronary intervention or surgery, who is having troublesome exertional angina despite combination treatment with a long-acting nitrate, beta blocker and calcium antagonist

230 ANTICOAGULANTS AND ANTIPLATELET DRUGS

A	Aspirin	G	Aspirin + clopidogrel
B	Warfarin	H	Aspirin + dipyridamole
C	Intravenous heparin	I	Aspirin + clopidogrel + subcutaneous enoxaparin
D	Subcutaneous enoxaparin		
E	Dipyridamole	J	Clopidogrel + dipyridamole
F	Clopidogrel		

Which drug or drug combination is appropriate for each of the following scenarios?

1 Treatment of a 68-year-old man with known ischaemic heart disease, admitted to hospital with unstable angina

2 Treatment of a 65-year-old woman, known to have mitral stenosis secondary to childhood rheumatic fever, who is otherwise well and presents with a two-week history of atrial fibrillation

3 Immediate treatment of a 30-year-old man, normally well, who presents with a suspected deep vein thrombosis following a long-haul flight

4 Immediate treatment of a 70-year-old woman, known to have pancreatic carcinoma and renal impairment (creatinine 300 μmol/L), who presents with a suspected deep vein thrombosis

5 Treatment of a 55-year-old man with known stable angina pectoris, on beta blocker treatment, who is allergic to aspirin

231 HEART FAILURE

A	Daunorubicin	F	Glyceryl trinitrate
B	Infliximab	G	Ibuprofen
C	Amlodipine	H	Verapamil
D	Digoxin	I	Amiloride
E	Bisoprolol	J	Furosemide

Link each of 1 to 5 below with the most appropriate item from A to J:

1 Improves survival in stable heart failure
2 Positive inotrope
3 Contraindicated in heart failure because a strong negative inotrope
4 Causes hypokalaemia
5 Cardiotoxic

232 CARDIAC DYSRHYTHMIAS

A	Intravenous adenosine	F	Intravenous digoxin
B	Intravenous lidocaine	G	Intravenous verapamil
C	Oral disopyramide	H	Oral mexiletine
D	Direct current cardioversion	I	Intravenous atropine
E	Oral sotalol	J	None of the above

Which of the above is appropriate for each clinical situation below?

1 Prevention of paroxysmal atrial fibrillation in an otherwise well 60-year-old man

2 Treatment of supraventricular tachycardia in a 28-year-old woman, otherwise well, where vagal manoeuvres have failed

3 Treatment of symptomatic supraventricular tachycardia in a 22-year-old woman with brittle asthma, where vagal manoeuvres have failed

4 Treatment of symptomatic sinus bradycardia (rate 35/minute) in a 62-year-old man with an acute inferior myocardial infarction

5 Treatment of frequent asymptomatic ventricular ectopic beats in a 65-year-old man with an acute anterior myocardial infarction

ANSWERS: see pages 97–100

ANSWERS

MCQ ANSWERS

169 a) True   Atheroma is the commonest cause of ischaemic heart
b) True   disease, stroke and peripheral vascular disease
c) True
d) True
e) True

170 a) True   The anion-exchange resins colestyramine and colestipol are
b) True   not absorbed into the systemic circulation and bind bile acids
c) False   in the gut lumen inhibiting reabsorption of bile salts and
d) False   cholesterol. They have been almost completely superseded
e) True   by statins in the management of hypercholesterolaemia.
Colestyramine causes malabsorption of fat-soluble
vitamins, and is used to treat pruritus in patients with
incomplete biliary obstruction. Side-effects include
flatulence, constipation and nausea

171 a) True   The fibrates stimulate lipoprotein lipase and reduce plasma
b) False   triglyceride. They also tend to reduce LDL cholesterol and to
c) False   raise HDL cholesterol. They can cause myositis which is
d) False   more common in alcoholics, patients with impaired renal
e) True   function and in patients on concurrent HMG-CoA
reductase inhibitors (statins). Other adverse effects include
nausea and abdominal discomfort

172 a) True   HMG-CoA reductase is the rate-limiting step in cholesterol
b) True   biosynthesis from acetate. HMG-CoA reductase inhibitors
c) False   are ineffective in rare patients with homozygous familial
d) True   hypercholesterolaemia as they cannot make LDL receptors.
e) False   – Ezetimibe is used in combination with diet and statins
for severe hypercholesterolaemia or when statins are
contraindicated

173 a) True   Although hypertension is usually 'essential' (i.e. idiopathic),
b) True   the possibility of secondary hypertension must always be
c) True   considered. Equally important is the confirmation or
d) True   rejection of persistent hypertension by repeated measures
e) True   (blood pressure is very variable) and the identification of
other treatable risk factors such as diabetes, smoking,
hypercholesterolaemia and obesity

174 a) True   Thiazide diuretics (e.g. bendroflumethiazide) remain
b) True   a logical first choice for treating older patients and

	c)	False
	d)	False
	e)	True

Afro-Caribbean patients with mild hypertension unless contraindicated by some co-existent disease, and are also valuable in patients with more severe hypertension in combination with other therapy

175 a) True
b) True
c) False
d) True
e) True

The relatively cardioselective β-adrenoreceptor antagonists, atenolol and metoprolol, are no longer used as first-line treatment of hypertension in the UK. They are particularly valuable in patients with additional pathology, such as angina or heart failure (e.g. metoprolol, carvedilol), or who have survived a myocardial infarction. Atenolol is a polar drug and undergoes renal elimination whilst metoprolol is non-polar and is metabolized by CYP450 2D6

176 a) True
b) True
c) False
d) False
e) False

Afro-Caribbean patients are less likely to have high circulating renin levels, hence beta blockers and ACE inhibitors are less likely to be effective. This difference is statistical and based on large populations. Both ACE inhibitors and beta blockers can be effective in individual Afro-Caribbean patients but a thiazide or calcium channel antagonist is usually the antihypertensive of first choice

177 a) True
b) True
c) False
d) False
e) False

ACE inhibitors inhibit the conversion of inactive angiotensin I to active angiotensin II, a powerful vasoconstrictor, and also inhibit the breakdown of the vasodilator peptides such as bradykinin. ACE inhibitors are of particular value in treating diabetic hypertensive patients as they significantly slow down the progressive renal impairment typical in these patients

178 a) False
b) False
c) True
d) True
e) False

Angiotensin-II receptor antagonists, unlike ACE inhibitors, do not inhibit the breakdown of bradykinin, hence dry cough is a much less common adverse effect. In bilateral renal artery stenosis glomerular filtration is dependant on angiotensin-II-mediated efferent arteriolar vasoconstriction

179 a) False
b) True
c) False
d) False
e) False

Nifedipine is used in the management of Raynaud's syndrome, hypertension and angina. Modified-release tablets are preferred. Amlodipine is a once-daily calcium channel blocker with similar pharmacodynamic properties

180 a) True
b) True
c) False
d) True
e) False

Nifedipine, unlike verapamil, has little effect on the conducting system of the heart. It can worsen angina due to a reflex tachycardia whilst verapamil causes a bradycardia. Both drugs are effective arterial dilators. Verapamil is a much more potent negative inotrope and has a greater inhibitory effect on intestinal peristalsis

181 a) True Non-specific alpha blockers such as phenoxybenzamine
b) False cause profound postural hypotension and reflex tachycardia.
c) True Doxazosin does not block presynaptic α_2 receptors that are
d) True normally stimulated by released noradrenaline and which
e) True inhibit further transmitter release. This is a negative
feedback pathway hence there is little reflex tachycardia
with doxazosin although first-dose hypotension is a
problem; therefore start with a low dose, usually at night

182 a) True Sodium nitroprusside is valuable in treating hypertensive
b) True encephalopathy and in the management of certain types of
c) False 'shock' when it is combined with positive inotropes.
d) True Continuous blood pressure monitoring is essential as it
e) True causes profound hypotension. It has a half-life of less than
10 minutes

183 a) True Although generally safe and not contraindicated in asthma
b) True and pregnancy, methyldopa is often poorly tolerated. The
c) True dose should be slowly titrated upwards. Drowsiness and
d) True fatigue may be intolerable when used chronically. It is a well
e) False recognized (but uncommon) cause of drug fever and
Coombs'-positive haemolytic anaemia

184 a) True Diuretics worsen symptoms of bladder neck obstruction,
b) True whereas α_1 antagonists improve such symptoms as well as
c) False synergizing with ACE inhibitors
d) False
e) True

185 a) True – More common in slow acetylators
b) True – Fluid retention is also a problem
c) True – Worse if on diuretics
d) False – May reduce tremor
e) False – First-dose hypotension can occur so use same precautions
as with an ACE inhibitor

186 a) False The highest concentration of oxygen available should be
b) True used unless there is coincident pulmonary disease with CO_2
c) True retention. Aspirin and opening the occluded artery (either
d) True with thrombolytic therapy or angioplasty) have an additive
e) False beneficial effect on reduction of infarct size and
improvement in survival. There is evidence of some benefit
from early treatment with ACE inhibitors post infarction in
patients with left ventricular dysfunction

187 a) True Patients with unstable angina require urgent admission,
b) True urgent antiplatelet therapy (aspirin and clopidogrel) plus

c) True
d) False
e) True

antithrombotic therapy (usually low molecular weight heparin). GTN (usually by infusion in this indication) is often effective in relieving pain, but does not significantly alter outcome

188 a) True
b) True
c) True
d) False
e) True

GTN is generally best used as acute prophylaxis (i.e. immediately before undertaking strenuous activity). The spray has a longer 'shelf-life' but is more expensive than the sublingual GTN. GTN is subject to extensive presystemic metabolism if swallowed. Longer-acting oral nitrates (e.g. isosorbide mononitrate) are effective as regular prophylactic therapy

189 a) False
b) True
c) True
d) False
e) True

Beta blockers slow the heart, are negatively inotropic (but metoprolol, bisoprolol, carvedilol and nebivolol may be of value in stable heart failure) and reduce arterial blood pressure, are antidysrhythmic, increase peripheral vascular resistance, reduce plasma renin activity and predispose to bronchoconstriction

190 a) True
b) True
c) False
d) False
e) True

Modifiable risk factors should be sought and attended to. Stopping smoking is particularly important. ACE inhibitors are recommended for patients with left ventricular dysfunction

191 a) True
b) True
c) False
d) False
e) False

In addition to hypertension and angina, verapamil is used to treat supraventricular tachycardia. Nimodipine helps prevent cerebral vasospasm and nifedipine is used in Raynaud's syndrome

192 a) True
b) True
c) True
d) True
e) False

The commonest side-effects of nifedipine and amlodipine are flushing and headache. They have no significant effect on the conduction system of the heart

193 a) True
b) True
c) True
d) False
e) False

Thromboxane (TX) A_2 is the main cyclo-oxygenase product of activated platelets and is proaggregatory and a vasoconstrictor

194 a) True
b) False
c) False
d) True
e) False

Streptokinase combines with plasminogen to form an activator complex that converts remaining free plasminogen to plasmin which dissolves fibrin. The potential benefit lessens with delay but the value of treatment within 24 hours is well established

195 a) False – Alteplase is a direct-acting plasminogen activator
 b) False – Immediate heparin following alteplase is necessary to prevent re-occlusion
 c) False
 d) True – Also indicated in acute myocardial infarction and acute ischaemic stroke (under specialist neurologists)
 e) False

196 a) True Immune reactions are important with streptokinase and its
 b) True prodrug anistreplase. It seems unlikely that mild infections
 c) False such as sore throats reduce its efficacy. 'Recent' dental
 d) True extraction is considered a contraindication
 e) False

197 a) True Unfractionated heparin binds to antithrombin III, the
 b) True naturally occurring inhibitor of thrombin and of the other
 c) True serine proteases (factors IXa, Xa and XIa), enormously
 d) True potentiating its inhibitory action
 e) True

198 a) False Prophylactic once-daily subcutaneous LMWH reduces the
 b) False risk of thromboembolism associated with major surgery.
 c) True Laboratory monitoring of coagulation is not necessary in
 d) True routine clinical use. The benefit normally outweighs the
 e) False increased risk of bleeding in major orthopaedic surgery

199 a) True The commonest adverse effect is bleeding. This can be
 b) True treated by stopping the infusion (if relevant), local
 c) True compression, protamine sulphate and, if severe and
 d) False continues in spite of the above, fresh frozen plasma
 e) False

200 a) True LMWH is preferred to heparin unless renal failure is
 b) True present
 c) True
 d) True – Fondaparinux, a synthetic pentasaccharide, has been shown to be superior to unfractionated heparin or LMWH for thromboprophylaxis in some studies
 e) True

201 a) True Warfarin is the most commonly prescribed oral
 b) True anticoagulant. It usually takes at least 3 days to achieve
 c) False adequate anticoagulation. If more rapid action is required
 d) True intravenous heparin and oral warfarin are used until the INR is in the usual therapeutic range (2–3 for most indications)
 e) True – Heparin only influences the INR if the APTT is >2.5 times the control. The laboratory can allow for this by the *in vitro* addition of protamine

202 a) True   Other contraindications include active bleeding, blood
    b) False   dyscrasias with haemorrhagic diatheses, dissecting
    c) True   aneurysm of the aorta and recent CNS surgery. Aspirin and
    d) False   warfarin should not be used together routinely, although
    e) False   trials of low-dose combination therapy are in progress

203 a) True   Warfarin has a narrow therapeutic range and steep
    b) True   dose–response curve. It is metabolized by CYP450.
    c) False   Cimetidine, an H_2 blocker used to reduce gastric acid
    d) False   production, and fluvoxamine, a selective serotonin reuptake
    e) False   inhibitor (SSRI) antidepressant, both inhibit CYP450.
    St John's wort, carbamazepine and smoking induce
    CYP450. The INR must be monitored to reduce both the
    risk of bleeding and inadequate anticoagulation

204 a) False   Thromboxane A_2 is synthesized by activated platelets and
    b) True   acts on platelet receptors to cause further activation and
    c) False   propagation of the aggregate. It also acts on vascular smooth
    d) True   muscle to cause vasoconstriction. Heparin inhibits thrombin,
    e) True   which is a platelet agonist, as well as causing coagulation

205 a) False   Clopidogrel is combined with aspirin to treat patients with
    b) True   acute coronary syndrome/myocardial infarction and
    c) False   following percutaneous coronary intervention with stent
    d) True   placement. It may be substituted for aspirin in other
    e) False   indications as an antiplatelet drug if aspirin is poorly
    tolerated

206 a) True   Prostacyclin may be used to prevent coagulation in
    b) True   extracorporeal circuits. It causes flushing, headache, reduced
    c) True   diastolic pressure, increased pulse pressure and usually a
    d) False   reflex tachycardia. Occasionally vagally mediated
    e) False   bradycardia and hypotension occur

207 a) False   The major influences on preload are blood volume and
    b) True   capacitance vessel tone
    c) False
    d) True
    e) False

208 a) True   Negative inotropes, direct cardiac toxins (e.g. daunorubicin)
    b) True   and drugs that cause salt retention (e.g. NSAIDs) aggravate
    c) True   heart failure. Excessive tachycardia does not allow
    d) True   sufficient time for the ventricle to fill in diastole
    e) False

209 a) False   In addition to helping relieve the acute anxiety and
    b) False   discomfort associated with acute pulmonary oedema, opioids

c) True   dilate capacitance vessels
d) True
e) True

210 **a)** True   Loop diuretics inhibit $Na^+/K^+/2Cl^-$ co-transport in the
      b) True   thick ascending limb of Henle's loop
      c) True
      d) True
      e) True

211 **a)** False   ACE inhibitors and angiotensin-II antagonists act as
      b) False   arterial and venous vasodilators in cardiac failure,
      c) False   prolonging survival
      d) True
      e) False

212 **a)** False   Spironolactone can cause life-threatening hyperkalaemia,
      b) True   however if renal function is not appreciably impaired
      c) False   and serum potassium monitored, the addition of
      d) False   spironolactone to the loop diuretic/ACE inhibitor
      e) True   combination is usually beneficial. Although beta blockers
              are negative inotropes, several trials have shown that
              careful addition of beta blockers to other treatments (e.g.
              ACE inhibitors) improve survival

213 **a)** True   Dobutamine is a positive inotrope used predominantly in
      b) True   cardiogenic shock. Hypovolaemia must be corrected before
      c) False   its use
      d) False
      e) True

214 **a)** False   The management of sinus tachycardia is directed to the
      b) True   underlying cause (e.g. pain, anxiety, left ventricular failure,
      c) True   asthma, thyrotoxicosis) and iatrogenic factors. Of calcium
      d) True   antagonists, verapamil causes bradycardia, dihyropyridines
      e) False   can cause reflex tachycardia, and diltiazem seldom causes
              appreciable changes in heart rate. Esmolol is a beta blocker
              with a very short duration of action

215 **a)** True   Lidocaine has a narrow therapeutic index but is used for the
      b) True   treatment of ventricular tachycardia and fibrillation (post DC
      c) False   cardioversion). It is also used as a local anaesthetic
      d) True
      e) False

216 **a)** True   A prolonged QT interval predisposes to torsade
      b) True   de pointes, a form of ventricular tachycardia
      c) True   – Used for cytomegalovirus (CMV) retinitis and patients
              with acquired immunodeficiency syndrome (AIDS)

d) True   – An immunosuppressant whose adverse effects include cardiomyopathy

e) True

217 a) True   Amiodarone, a class III agent, is highly effective in both
b) True   supraventricular and ventricular arrhythmias. It is not a
c) False   negative inotrope in contrast to most antidysrhythmic
d) True   agents
e) True

218 a) True   Adverse effects are many and varied and are common
b) True   when plasma amiodarone concentration exceeds 2.5 mg/L.
c) True   Most are reversible on stopping treatment, but this is not true
d) True   of pulmonary fibrosis
e) True

219 a) True   Amiodarone is highly protein bound and is slowly excreted
b) True   by the liver. Antidysrhythmic activity may persist for several
c) False   months after stopping treatment
d) True
e) True

220 a) True   Sotalol is a β-adrenoreceptor antagonist (class II) with
b) False   additional class III antidysrhythmic activity
c) True
d) True
e) False

221 a) True   Verapamil slows intracardiac conduction affecting in
b) True   particular the atrioventricular (AV) node but also the
c) True   sinoatrial (SA) node. It is a potent negative inotrope. It
d) False   should be avoided in WPW as it can increase conduction
e) False   through an accessory pathway

222 a) False   Adenosine is used to terminate supraventricular tachycardia
b) False   (SVT). It is particularly useful diagnostically in patients with
c) False   regular broad complex tachycardia which is suspected of
d) True   being SVT with aberrant conduction. If adenosine terminates
e) True   the bradycardia the AV node is involved

223 a) True   The main use of digoxin as an antidysrhythmic is to control
b) True   the ventricular rate (and hence improve cardiac output) in
c) False   patients with atrial fibrillation. Drugs causing hypokalaemia
d) True   aggravate digoxin toxicity
e) False

224 a) True   Isoprenaline, a beta agonist, is likely to be dysrhythmogenic
b) False   and will increase myocardial oxygen consumption.

c) False
d) False
e) False

Verapamil is a potent negative inotrope and is only effective in SVT

225
a) False
b) False
c) False
d) False
e) True

Bradycardia and first-degree heart block are common post inferior myocardial infarction. If the bradycardia causes symptoms 0.6 mg atropine intravenously is usually effective

226
a) False
b) True
c) False
d) False
e) False

If causing immediate cardiovascular embarrassment, DC cardioversion is indicated in ventricular tachycardia. Otherwise, if intravenous lidocaine is ineffective, or oral prophylaxis is required, amiodarone may be used. Intravenous magnesium sulphate has been recommended for torsades de pointes. It also has a major role in eclampsia for the prevention of recurrent seizures

EMQ ANSWERS

227 ATHEROMA AND THROMBOSIS

1 J Ezetimibe blocks cholesterol absorption and is useful when combined with a statin. (Specialists sometimes combine fibrates with statins but this is not routine as there is an increased risk of adverse effects.)

2 D Epoprostenol (prostacyclin) is used to inhibit platelet aggregation during haemodialysis. It can also be used in primary pulmonary hypertension.

3 F Fenofibrate, bezafibrate and gemfibrozil are used mainly for patients with mixed dyslipidaemia with severely raised triglycerides, especially if they are poorly responsive to statins.

4 H Colestyramine used to be combined with a statin but has been rendered largely obsolete by ezetimibe because of its inconvenience and adverse effects. Colestyramine is indicated for pruritus associated with partial biliary obstruction and primary biliary cirrhosis, diarrhoea associated with Crohn's disease, ileal resection, vagotomy, diabetic vagal neuropathy and radiation.

5 A Simvastatin is very well tolerated but myalgia is its most common adverse effect (see *Textbook of Clinical Pharmacology and Therapeutics*, Chapter 27).

228 HYPERTENSION

See *Textbook of Clinical Pharmacology and Therapeutics*, Chapter 28.

1 J Thiazide diuretics are associated with erectile dysfunction which is reversible on stopping the thiazide. Calcium channel blockers (e.g. amlodipine) and thiazide diuretics are the antihypertensives of first choice in Afro-Caribbean patients.

2 C Doxazosin has postsynaptic α_1-blocking activity and is an effective hypotensive agent. First-dose hypotension is a potential problem. It relaxes smooth muscle in benign prostatic hyperplasia improving flow rate and reducing obstructive symptoms.

3 F Spironolactone competes with aldosterone for its intracellular receptors. Its indications include Conn's syndrome, secondary hyperaldosteronism in ascites and resistant, low renin hypertension. Hyperkalaemia is a potential problem, particularly if on another potassium-sparing drug (e.g. an ACE inhibitor such as trandolapril), or if there is renal impairment.

4 G Candesartan is an angiotensin II blocker. Unlike ACE inhibitors it does not inhibit the breakdown of bradykinin, the likely cause of an ACE inhibitor-induced cough.

5 I Although not sinister, ankle oedema is a troublesome adverse effect of calcium channel blockers (less common with verapamil). Thiazides are often effective in Afro-Caribbean patients. Metabolic adverse effects include hypokalaemia, hyperglycaemia, hypercalcaemia and hyperuricaemia.

229 ISCHAEMIC HEART DISEASE

1 D Sublingual GTN is an effective and convenient acute treatment for angina.

2 C Recombinant tissue plasminogen activator (alteplase) is an effective thrombolytic.

3 A Long-term use of ACE inhibitors (e.g. ramipril) post myocardial infarction in patients with left ventricular dysfunction prevents cardiac remodelling and subsequent worsening of heart failure.

4 I Numerous large studies have shown statins to be beneficial in reducing future cardiac events in this situation.

5 H Nicorandil combines activation of the potassium K_{ATP} channel with vasodilator (nitric oxide donor) actions.

230 ANTICOAGULANTS AND ANTIPLATELET DRUGS

1 **I** Aspirin + clopidogrel + subcutaneous enoxaparin (an LMWH) approximately halves the likelihood of myocardial infarction in patients with acute coronary syndrome.

2 **B** Warfarin would reduce the risk of stroke in this patient with mitral stenosis and atrial fibrillation.

3 **D** Subcutaneous enoxaparin is an effective and convenient (once-daily subcutaneous injection) acute treatment in suspected deep vein thrombosis.

4 **C** Unfractionated heparin has been replaced by LMWH for most indications but remains important in patients with impaired or rapidly changing renal function.

5 **F** Clopidogrel is an inactive prodrug that is converted in the liver to an active metabolite that binds to and irreversibly inhibits platelet ADP receptors, thereby inhibiting platelet aggregation and arterial thrombotic disease.

231 HEART FAILURE

Heart failure occurs when the heart fails to deliver adequate oxygenated blood to the tissues during exercise, or in severe cases, at rest.

1 **E** Bisoprolol, and other β-adrenoreceptor antagonists, although negative inotropes can improve survival in heart failure, if the dose is titrated carefully. This improvement is probably through antagonism of counter-regulatory sympathetic activation.

2 **D** Digoxin inhibits Na^+/K^+ ATPase causing an increase in intracellular Ca^{2+} which results in a positive inotropic effect, although its main value is in reducing ventricular rate in rapid atrial fibrillation.

3 **H** Verapamil is a strong negative inotrope.

4 **J** Furosemide, a loop diuretic, causes hypokalaemia which predisposes to dysrhythmias.

5 **A** Daunorubicin, ethanol, imatinib, gefitinib and trastuzumab are cardiac toxins.

232 CARDIAC DYSRHYTHMIAS

1 **E** Sotalol is a β-adrenoreceptor antagonist which additionally has substantial class III activity.

2 **A** Intravenous adenosine is used to terminate SVT. Adenosine A_1 receptors block AV nodal conduction.

3 **G** Intravenous verapamil is used to terminate SVT in patients who are not haemodynamically compromised if adenosine is contraindicated. Verapamil is a calcium channel blocker.

4 **I** Atropine, a selective antagonist of acetylcholine at muscarinic receptors, accelerates the heart rate by inhibiting vagal tone.

5 **J** Asymptomatic ventricular ectopic beats post anterior myocardial infarction do not require any drug therapy. Trials of anti-dysrhythmic drugs in this situation have shown that they are more likely to increase mortality.

CHAPTER FIVE

RESPIRATORY SYSTEM

MULTIPLE CHOICE QUESTIONS

233 The following should be administered to an otherwise healthy 27-year-old male with acute severe asthma:

a) Intravenous midazolam
b) Nebulized salbutamol
c) Intravenous glucocorticosteroids
d) Nebulized salmeterol
e) Continuous high percentage oxygen (FiO_2 35–40 per cent)

234 Beta$_2$ agonists (e.g. salbutamol, terbutaline, salmeterol):

a) Relax bronchial smooth muscle
b) Inhibit release of mast cell and other inflammatory mediators
c) Reduce heart rate
d) Cause pulmonary vasoconstriction
e) Decrease intracellular cyclic adenosine monophosphate (cAMP)

235 Pharmacodyamic properties of salmeterol include:

a) Tremor
b) Exacerbation of atrial dysrhythmias
c) Hyperkalaemia
d) Prolonged pharmacodynamic effects allowing twice-daily dosing
e) Seizures

236 Omalizumab:

a) Is contraindicated in patients with IgE-mediated sensitivity to inhaled allergen
b) Is used to treat severe acute attacks
c) Is administered by subcutaneous injection
d) Inhibits warfarin metabolism via CYP 2C9
e) Cannot be used in children

237 Ipratropium bromide:

a) Is administered intravenously

b) Causes bronchodilatation because of its antagonistic effects at the cholinergic M_2/M_3 receptors

c) Has a more rapid onset of bronchodilatation than beta$_2$ agonists

d) Has a bitter taste

e) May precipitate glaucoma in high doses

238 Adverse effects associated with the use of theophylline include:

a) Cardiac dysrhythmias

b) Convulsions

c) Oral candidiasis

d) Headache

e) Nausea and vomiting

239 In acute severe asthma hydrocortisone:

a) Is usually given via the intravenous route

b) Subjective improvement following steroid administration takes 30–60 minutes

c) Is contraindicated in growing children

d) Is contraindicated in pregnancy

e) Should not be administered until at least two doses of nebulized salbutamol have been administered without significant evidence of sustained bronchodilatation

240 Administration of fluticasone via a metered dose inhaler:

a) Allows reduction in the maintenance dose of oral prednisolone in chronic asthma

b) More of the dose is swallowed than enters the lungs

c) Does not cause hypothalamo-pituitary-adrenal suppression at a dose of 2000 μg/day

d) Has a lower systemic bioavailability than beclomethasone

e) In children, causes reversible inhibition of long bone growth at high doses

241 Inhaled sodium cromoglicate:

a) Is effective in alleviating an acute episode of allergic asthma

b) Has no benefit in preventing exercise-induced bronchospasm

c) Prevents antigen–antibody combination

d) Inhibits mediator release from mast cells

e) Causes cardiac dysrhythmias by prolonging the QTc

242 Montelukast:

a) Is a competitive antagonist at the Cys LT_1 receptor
b) Can be given orally
c) Is usually taken once daily at bedtime
d) May be associated with Churg–Strauss syndrome
e) Is not beneficial to patients with antigen-induced asthma

243 The following drugs can produce pulmonary fibrosis:

a) Methotrexate
b) Bleomycin
c) Busulphan
d) Lisinopril
e) Amiodarone

244 Pulmonary eosinophilia is caused by the following drugs:

a) Methysergide
b) Aspirin
c) Nitrofurantoin
d) Carmustine (BCNU)
e) Sulfasalazine

245 The following agents if given to an asthmatic are likely to cause catastrophic bronchospasm:

a) Carvedilol
b) Losartan
c) Adenosine
d) Lidocaine (lignocaine)
e) Bethanecol

246 The following drugs are used as 'standard of care' when treating a patient with type II (hypoxic–hypercanic) respiratory failure:

a) 35 per cent oxygen
b) Doxapram
c) Salbutamol
d) Methylprednisolone
e) Dantrolene

Answers: see pages 105–107

EXTENDED MATCHING QUESTIONS

247 RESPIRATORY DRUGS – MECHANISM OF ACTION

A	Salbutamol	F	Sodium cromoglicate
B	Salmeterol	G	Theophylline
C	Tiotropium	H	Omalizumab
D	Methylprednisolone	I	Cetirizine
E	Montelukast	J	Zafirlukast

Select the drug whose mechanism of action is described below:

1 Inhibits transcription of proinflammatory cytokines
2 Binds to the Fc portion of IgE
3 Inhibits H_1 but not H_2 receptors
4 Modulates the firing of respiratory C fibres
5 Competitively inhibits M_2 and M_3 muscarinic receptors

248 RESPIRATORY DRUGS – ADVERSE EFFECTS

A	Terbutaline	F	Nedocromil
B	Formoterol	G	Theophylline
C	Azithromycin	H	Omalizumab
D	Dexamethasone	I	Loratadine
E	Montelukast	J	Codeine

Select the drugs most frequently associated with the adverse effects described below:

1 Seizures
2 Apnoea
3 QTc prolongation
4 Hypertension
5 Anaphylaxis

ANSWERS: see page 108

ANSWERS

MCQ ANSWERS

233 a) False   Never give anxiolytics/sedatives in acute asthma.
   b) True   Intravenous fluids are administered to correct/prevent
   c) True   dehydration. Antibiotics are administered if there is
   d) False   history/signs of infection. Refractory cases require an
   e) True   intravenous short-acting beta$_2$ agonist (salbutamol) or as a
last resort theophylline. If these are inadequate,
intermittent positive pressure ventilation is required.
Nebulized salmeterol is not available and its onset of
bronchodilation is too slow to be used acutely

234 a) True   Beta$_2$ agonists stimulate the β_2 receptor which via linked
   b) True   G-proteins increases adenylyl cyclase activity and increases
   c) False   intracellular cAMP. They cause a tachycardia and
   d) False   vasodilatation
   e) False

235 a) True   Beta$_2$ agonists are generally well tolerated when given by
   b) True   inhalation. Salmeterol, a long-acting beta$_2$ agonist, is
   c) False   inhaled twice daily and reduces the need for shorter-acting
   d) True   agents and possibly the dose of inhaled corticosteroids.
   e) False   Beta$_2$ agonists cause hypokalaemia

236 a) False   Omalizumab is a recombinant humanized IgG$_1$ monoclonal
   b) False   anti-IgE antibody. It is used in paediatric patients (12 or
   c) True   older) who have allergic/atopic asthma refractory to
   d) False   maximal regular therapy. If there is no improvement in 16
   e) False   weeks it should be discontinued, see NICE guidelines 2007

237 a) False   Inhaled antimuscarinic drugs such as ipratropium and
   b) True   tiotropium (long acting once daily) are effective as acute
   c) False   and maintenance bronchodilator therapy in asthma. Their
   d) True   action is slower in onset than that of beta$_2$ agonists. High
   e) True   doses usually via a nebulizer may precipitate acute
glaucoma or urinary retention

238 a) True   Theophylline has a narrow therapeutic index and its
   b) True   pharmacokinetics show considerable interindividual
   c) False   variation. Because of hepatic metabolism it is prone to a
   d) True   number of drug–drug interactions which may lead to
   e) True   toxicity (see Table 3). Its main side-effects are
gastrointestinal, cardiovascular and CNS

Table 3 Factors influencing theophylline clearance

Factors decreasing theophylline clearance and suggested initial dose* adjustment (assuming normal dose is 100%)	Factors increasing theophylline clearance and suggested initial dose* adjustment (assuming normal dose is 100%)
Congestive cardiac failure (40%)	Hyperthyroidism (150%)
Hepatic disease, cirrhosis (40%)	Marijuana (150%)
Neonates (60%)	Smoking (150%)
Pneumonia (70%)	Charcoal barbecued meat (130%)
Old age (80%)	
Drugs	Drugs
Azole-antifungals	Carbamazepine (150%)
(e.g. ketoconazole etc.) (50%)	Phenytoin (150%)
Cimetidine (50%)	Rifampicin (150%)
Fluoroquinolones	High protein, low carbohydrate
(e.g. ciprofloxacin) (50%)	diet (150%)
Chloramphenicol (75%)	Ethanol (chronic) (120%)
Erythromycin (75%)	
Flu vaccine and interferon (75%)	
Propranolol (70%)	

*Subsequent dose adjustment to be made in the light of plasma concentration monitoring, which should be carried out more frequently in the circumstances listed. The suggested adjustments are obviously very approximate, and depend on the extent of exposure to the various agents.

239 a) True
b) False
c) False
d) False
e) False

Objective improvement does not occur until 6 hours and is maximal 13 hours after the start of intravenous glucocorticosteroid treatment in asthma. This delay is due to the pharmacodynamics of glucocorticoids which work via modifying transcription of certain genes and thus affecting their protein synthesis. They should be administered early in acute asthma

240 a) True
b) True
c) False
d) False
e) True

Systemic adverse events are rarely significant with inhaled glucocorticoids unless the dose exceeds e.g. 1000 μg of fluticasone or its equivalent. They are invaluable in the prophylaxis of asthma and have been shown to reduce asthma deaths and exacerbations in patients with chronic obstructive pulmonary disease (COPD)

241 a) False
b) False
c) False

Sodium cromoglicate is administered by inhalation of a powder. Used prophylactically it can prevent type I and type III allergic reactions and exercise-induced asthma.

d) True   It is very safe although approximately 1:10 000 experience a
e) False   cough or hoarseness

242 a) True   It is a potent, oral, once-daily inhibitor of cysteinyl
    b) True   leukotrienes at the Cys LT_1 receptor. Thus its main action is
    c) True   to antagonize the potent proinflammatory effects of
    d) True   leukotrienes. It causes about a 5–10 per cent increase in
    e) False baseline FEV_1 but this takes about 1 hour to manifest. About
             5 per cent of patients develop a reversible transaminitis

243 a) True   Several cytotoxics, particularly if given with or following
    b) True   radiation, cause a severe pulmonary fibrosis that may not
    c) True   be reversible. Angiotensin-converting enzyme (ACE)
    d) False inhibitors – but not the angiotensin II receptor blockers
    e) True   (ARBs)) are associated with a dose-dependent chronic dry
             cough thought to be related to bradykinin accumulation

244 a) False Methysergide causes retroperitoneal fibrosis. Aspirin
    b) True   (and nitrofurantoin, imipramine, isoniazid, penicillins,
    c) True   sulfonamides and streptomycin) has been associated with
    d) False pulmonary eosinophilia. Carmustine causes pulmonary
    e) True   fibrosis

245 a) True   – Carvedilol is a non-selective beta blocker whose
             indications include hypertension, angina and, as adjunct
             to other agents, symptomatic chronic heart failure. The
             initial dose for this indication is a quarter of the other
             indications
    b) False
    c) True   – Adenosine causes bronchoconstriction by stimulating
             adenosine receptors
    d) False
    e) True   – Bethanecol and carbachol are acetylcholine analogues and
             increase cholinergic (parasympathetic) tone

246 a) False – Use low FiO_2 (e.g. 22–24 per cent) and titrate upwards
             based on blood gas response/clinical response
    b) False – Analeptics are no longer used unless mechanical
             ventilation is unavailable or contraindicated
    c) True
    d) True
    e) False – Dantrolene is a muscle relaxant; this would worsen
             respiratory failure

EMQ ANSWERS

247 RESPIRATORY DRUGS – MECHANISM OF ACTION

1 **D** Corticosteroids bind to its receptor in the cytoplasm, which then moves to the nucleus where it binds to DNA suppressing the transcription of certain genes such as interleukins and tumour necrosis factor (TNF) and enhancing transcription of $beta_2$ receptors, ACE and other anti-inflammatory entities.

2 **H** Omalizumab binds to the Fc receptor portion of IgE and blocks IgE, interacting with its receptor on inflammatory cells and reduces circulating IgE concentrations.

3 **I** Second-generation antihistamines are competitive antagonists at the H_1 receptor without significant binding to other receptors including the gastric H_2, muscarinic and serotonin receptors.

4 **F** Sodium cromoglicate – whose precise anti-inflammatory mechanism is not clearly defined modulates the firing of cough C fibres.

5 **C** Tiotropium is a competitive antagonist at respiratory muscarinic receptors and blocks parasympathetic effects on bronchiolar smooth muscle.

248 RESPIRATORY DRUGS – ADVERSE EFFECTS

1 **G** Theophylline adverse effects are usually dose (concentration) dependent with mainly gastrointestinal disturbances at low toxic concentrations, then CVS (dysrhythmias etc.) at moderately toxic concentrations and CNS stimulation at high toxic concentrations.

2 **J** Opiates are µ agonists and directly suppress the respiratory centre, leading to apnoea.

3 **B** Formoterol like other long-acting $beta_2$ agonists prolongs QTc and can also cause hypokalaemia which can exacerbate QTc prolongation.

4 **D** Corticosteroids in anti-inflammatory systemic doses cause an increase in vascular resistance and sodium retention which both lead to an increase in blood pressure.

5 **H** Omalizumab is a recombinant humanized monoclonal antibody to IgE, but as with all monoclonals can cause severe acute and delayed anaphylactic reactions. (It has a long terminal elimination half-life of approximately 21 days.)

ALIMENTARY SYSTEM

249 The following stimulate gastric acid secretion:
a) Vagal stimulation
b) Gastrin
c) Acetylcholine stimulation of the M_1 receptor
d) Histamine stimulation of the H_2 receptor
e) Increased intracellular cyclic adenosine monophosphate (cAMP)

250 Prostaglandin E_2:
a) Is the principal prostaglandin synthesized in the stomach
b) Stimulates gastric acid secretion
c) Causes vasoconstriction of submucosal blood vessels
d) Biosynthesis is inhibited by aspirin
e) Biosynthesis is inhibited by rectal indometacin

251 *Helicobacter pylori*:
a) Is strongly linked to the development of carcinoma of the colon
b) Is a bacterium that is strongly linked to the development and recurrence of peptic ulcer disease
c) Is usually found in the gastric antrum
d) Is uncommon in asymptomatic patients
e) Colonization of the stomach is inhibited by corticosteroids

252 The following accelerate healing in gastric ulcers:
a) Diclofenac
b) Stopping smoking
c) Corticosteroids
d) Ranitidine
e) Sucralfate

253 Antacids:

a) Large doses heal gastric ulcers more frequently than duodenal ulcers
b) Standard doses reduce gastric acidity for approximately 4 hours
c) Magnesium salts tend to cause diarrhoea
d) Aluminium salts tend to cause a diuresis
e) Magnesium and aluminium salts reduce the rate and extent of absorption of phenytoin

254 Cimetidine therapy is associated with:

a) Transient increase in serum prolactin
b) Irreversible gynaecomastia
c) Mental confusion in the elderly
d) Asystole after rapid intravenous injection
e) Reversible rise in serum creatinine

255 Eradication of *H. pylori* following a positive breath test is recommended in the following situations:

a) Duodenal ulcer
b) Gastric ulcer
c) Patients requiring long-term proton pump inhibitor treatment
d) Severe gastritis
e) Mucosa-associated lymphoid tissue lymphoma

256 In comparison to cimetidine, ranitidine:

a) Does not bind to androgen receptors
b) Is less likely to cause gynaecomastia
c) Penetrates the blood–brain barrier to a lesser extent
d) Is not available for parenteral use
e) Has a lower affinity for CYP450

257 Omeprazole:

a) Is an irreversible inhibitor of the hydrogen/potassium adenosine triphosphatase locus of the gastric parietal cell
b) Reduces gastric acid secretion
c) Is the drug of choice in Zollinger–Ellison syndrome
d) Has a plasma half-life of approximately 1 hour
e) Requires dose reduction in renal failure

258 Omeprazole enhances the effects of the following drugs through inhibition of drug metabolism:

a) Atenolol
b) Amoxicillin
c) Captopril
d) Warfarin
e) Phenytoin

259 Problems associated with proton pump inhibitors include:
  a) Masking symptoms of gastric cancer
  b) Diarrhoea, nausea and vomiting
  c) Increased risk of gastrointestinal infection
  d) Headache
  e) Prolonged QT interval on ECG

260 Misoprostol:
  a) Is a synthetic analogue of prostaglandin E
  b) Inhibits cyclo-oxygenase
  c) Causes vasodilatation in the submucosa
  d) Is rapidly and nearly completely absorbed
  e) Is contraindicated in pregnancy

261 Bismuth chelate (tripotassium dicitratobismuthate):
  a) Precipitates at acid pH
  b) Stimulates mucus production
  c) Has a direct toxic effect on *H. pylori*
  d) Causes pale stools
  e) Causes nausea

262 Sucralfate:
  a) Requires systemic absorption for anti-ulcer activity
  b) Contains aluminium
  c) Is effective in healing gastric ulcers
  d) Is contraindicated in pregnancy
  e) Is associated with constipation

263 The following drugs are used to prevent motion sickness:
  a) Hyoscine
  b) Promethazine
  c) Cinnarizine
  d) Metoclopramide
  e) Chlorpromazine

264 Cyclizine:
  a) Is a dopamine receptor antagonist
  b) Is effective in morphine-induced vomiting
  c) Is a proven teratogen
  d) Causes dry mouth
  e) Causes drowsiness

265 Metoclopramide:

a) Is most effective in centrally mediated vomiting
b) Is ineffective in drug-induced nausea
c) Increases the rate of gastric emptying
d) Should be avoided for 3–4 days following gastrointestinal surgery
e) High doses block $5HT_3$ receptors

266 Ondansetron:

a) Is a phenothiazine
b) Is not absorbed after oral administration
c) Is effective in preventing nausea and vomiting due to cancer chemotherapy and radiotherapy
d) Is ineffective in ciplastin-induced nausea
e) 1 per cent of patients have dystonic reactions

267 In ulcerative colitis:

a) Intravenous hydrocortisone is of proven value in the treatment of acute colitis
b) Oral corticosteroids are first line for maintenance treatment
c) Localized rectal disease often responds to prednisolone enemas/suppositories
d) In severe colitis codeine should be used
e) Fibre is contraindicated

268 Sulfasalazine:

a) Is a prodrug
b) Is used for maintenance treatment of ulcerative colitis
c) Is effective in small bowel Crohn's disease
d) Should be avoided in glucose 6-phosphate dehydrogenase (G6PD) deficiency
e) Should be avoided in salicylate hypersensitivity

269 Adverse effects associated with sulfasalazine include:

a) Blood dyscrasias
b) Oligospermia
c) Stevens–Johnson syndrome
d) Systemic lupus erythematosus (SLE)-like syndrome
e) Hepatitis

270 Mesalazine:

a) Is a prodrug consisting of a dimer of two 5-aminosalicylic acid molecules
b) Dissolves at the pH found in the terminal ileum and colon
c) Is contraindicated in sulphonamide hypersensitivity
d) Is associated with oligospermia
e) Is associated with interstitial nephritis

271 Infliximab:
- **a)** Inhibits tumour necrosis factor (TNF)
- **b)** Can only be administered on one occasion due to antibody production
- **c)** Is licensed for management of irritable bowel syndrome
- **d)** Can be used for maintenance therapy in Crohn's disease and ulcerative colitis
- **e)** Should not be used in a patient who has been treated with corticosteroids within the previous 12 months

272 The following drugs cause constipation:
- **a)** Amiodarone
- **b)** Amitriptyline
- **c)** Amoxicillin
- **d)** Misoprostol
- **e)** Metformin

273 Lactulose:
- **a)** Is a chemical stimulant to the colon
- **b)** Produces its effect 10–12 hours after an oral dose
- **c)** Requires colonic bacteria for activity
- **d)** Should not be administered concurrently with bran
- **e)** Is contraindicated in liver failure

274 Loperamide:
- **a)** Decreases intestinal transit time
- **b)** Increases bulk of gut contents
- **c)** Requires systemic absorption for activity on the bowel
- **d)** Causes pupil constriction
- **e)** Causes hypersalivation

275 Treatment of hepatic encephalopathy includes:
- **a)** Dietary protein restriction
- **b)** Emptying the lower bowel
- **c)** Oral lactulose
- **d)** Prophylactic vitamin K
- **e)** Oral methionine

276 The emergency drug therapy of portal hypertension and oesophageal varices may include:
- **a)** Terlipressin
- **b)** Chenodeoxycholic acid
- **c)** Calcitonin
- **d)** Octreotide
- **e)** Isoprenaline

277 The following drugs are associated with cholestatic jaundice/hepatitis:
   a) Ondansetron
   b) Methotrexate
   c) Synthetic oestrogens
   d) Chlorpromazine
   e) Rifampicin

278 The following are licensed in the UK for the management of obesity:
   a) Orlistat
   b) Sibutramine
   c) Thiazide diuretics
   d) Pizotifen
   e) Dexamphetamine

279 Rimonabant:
   a) Inhibits insulin secretion
   b) Systemic absorption is minimal
   c) Has been associated with pulmonary hypertension
   d) Is contraindicated in, and may cause, depression
   e) Is metabolized by CYP3A4

Answers: see pages 116–120

EXTENDED MATCHING QUESTIONS

280 ALIMENTARY SYSTEM

A	Gemcitabine	F	Ondansetron
B	Capecitabine	G	Olsalazine
C	Etoposide	H	Lansoprazole
D	Adefovir dipivoxil	I	Mebeverine
E	Loperamide	J	Ribavarin and peginterferon alfa

Match the drug from the list above with the mode of action/indication below:

1   Serotonin ($5HT_3$) receptor blockade
2   Symptomatic treatment of acute diarrhoea
3   Maintenance of remission of ulcerative colitis
4   Chemotherapy for patients with advanced or metastatic adenocarcinoma of the pancreas
5   Chronic hepatitis C

ANSWERS: see page 121

ANSWERS

MCQ ANSWERS

249 **a)** True   See Fig. 2
b) True
c) True
d) True
e) True

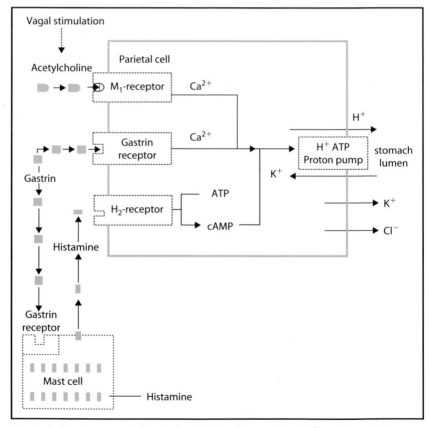

Fig. 2 Mechanisms regulating hydrochloric acid secretion. Ca^{2+}, calcium; ATP, adenosine triphosphate; cAMP, cyclic adenosine monophosphate; K^+, potassium; Cl^-, chloride

250 a) True   Prostaglandin E_2 is an important gastroprotective mediator.
    b) False   It inhibits secretion of acid, promotes secretion of protective
    c) False   mucus and causes vasodilation of submucosal blood
    d) True   vessels
    e) True

251 a) False   *Helicobacter pylori* is strongly linked to the development
    b) True   and recurrence of duodenal ulcer. Possible linkage to
    c) True   gastric carcinoma is under investigation
    d) False
    e) False

252 a) False   – Non-steroidal anti-inflammatory drug (NSAID),
                      ulcerogenic
    b) True   – More effective in preventing recurrence of duodenal ulcers
                      than H_2 blockers
    c) False   – Ulcerogenic
    d) True   – H_2 blocker
    e) True

253 a) False   Antacids are available without prescription and produce
    b) False   prompt but transient pain relief in patients with peptic
    c) True   ulceration. Aluminium salts cause constipation
    d) False
    e) True

254 a) True   Chronic cimetidine therapy causes reversible
    b) False   gynaecomastia in 0.1–0.2 per cent of patients. It is
    c) True   generally well tolerated. Cimetidine blocks the tubular
    d) True   secretion of creatinine
    e) True

255 a) True   Eradication should be confirmed, preferably by urea breath
    b) True   test at a minimum of four weeks post treatment
    c) True
    d) True
    e) True

256 a) True   All the H_2-receptor blockers currently available in the UK are
    b) True   effective in peptic ulceration and are well tolerated. There
    c) True   is most experience with cimetidine and ranitidine
    d) False
    e) True

257 a) True   Omeprazole, a proton pump inhibitor, is effective in
    b) True   reducing gastric acid secretion and in spite of its short half-life
    c) True   only has to be administered once daily since it acts
    d) True   irreversibly
    e) False

258 a) False   For drugs such as phenytoin and warfarin which have a
    b) False   narrow therapeutic index this is clinically significant
    c) False
    d) True
    e) True

259 a) True   There are currently five proton pump inhibitors licensed in
    b) True   the UK: esomeprazole, omeprazole, lansoprazole,
    c) True   pantoprazole and rabeprazole
    d) True
    e) False

260 a) True   Misoprostol inhibits gastric acid secretion, causes
    b) False   vasodilatation in the submucosa and stimulates production
    c) True   of protective mucus. It contracts uterine muscle and causes
    d) True   abortion
    e) True

261 a) True   Several studies show bismuth chelate to be as active as
    b) True   cimetidine in the healing of duodenal and gastric ulcers
    c) True   after 4–8 weeks of treatment. It is, however, associated with
    d) False   frequent minor adverse effects. Ranitidine bismuth chelate can
    e) True   be substituted for a proton pump inhibitor as part of 'triple
    therapy' for the eradication of *H. pylori*

262 a) False   Sucralfate, a basic aluminium salt, becomes a sticky
    b) True   adherent paste in the presence of acid which retains antacid
    c) True   efficacy and apparently coats the floor of ulcer craters
    d) False
    e) True

263 a) True   – Muscarinic antagonist; NB: anticholinergic side-effects
    b) True   – H_1 blocker minor antimuscarinic action
    c) True   – H_1 blocker minor antimuscarinic action
    d) False   – Dopamine receptor antagonist
    e) False   – Chlorpromazine is not used for motion sickness

264 a) False   Cyclizine is an H_1 blocker with additional antimuscarinic
    b) True   actions. Its indications are nausea, vomiting, vertigo,
    c) False   motion sickness and labyrinthine disorders
    d) True
    e) True

265 a) False   – Relatively ineffective in motion sickness and other forms of
    centrally mediated vomiting
    b) False
    c) True   – Increases the rate of absorption of oral drugs
    d) True
    e) True   – Effective in some patients in preventing cisplatin-induced
    nausea and vomiting

266 a) False – Ondansetron is a highly selective $5HT_3$-receptor antagonist
  b) False – Is used orally, rectally and intravenously
  c) True
  d) False
  e) False – Causes constipation

267 a) True – Correction of dehydration, nutritional and electrolyte imbalance are life-saving
  b) False – Because of side-effects
  c) True – Some systemic absorption may occur
  d) False – May precipitate paralytic ileus and megacolon
  e) False – A high-fibre diet and bulk-forming drugs are useful in adjusting faecal consistency

268 a) True – Broken down to 5-aminosalicylate and sulfapyridine
  b) True
  c) False
  d) True
  e) True

269 a) True   Adverse effects are more common in slow acetylators. Any
  b) True   patient who is receiving aminosalicylates must be advised
  c) True   to report unexplained bleeding, bruising, purpura or
  d) True   malaise
  e) True

270 a) False – This describes olsalazine
  b) True
  c) False – But is contraindicated in salicylate hypersensitivity
  d) False
  e) True – Contraindicated in renal impairment

271 a) True   Infliximab, a monoclonal antibody which inhibits TNF, is
  b) False   licensed for the management of severe active Crohn's
  c) False   disease and moderate to severe ulcerative colitis in patients
  d) True   who are refractory to or intolerant of corticosteroids and
  e) False   conventional immunosuppressants

272 a) True   The cause of any change in bowel habit should be
  b) True   determined before laxatives are used
  c) False
  d) False
  e) False

273 a) False   Lactulose is a disaccharide which is broken down in the
  b) False   colon by bacteria to unabsorbed organic anions which
  c) True   retain fluid in the gut lumen
  d) False
  e) False

274 a) False   See *Textbook of Clinical Pharmacology and Therapeutics*,
b) False   Chapter 34. Loperamide rarely causes CNS effects.
c) False   However, co-administration with quinidine, a known
d) False   inhibitor of the P-glycoprotein transmembrane pump, is
e) False   associated with respiratory depression independent of
changes in plasma concentration indicating increased
CNS penetration

275 a) True   See *Textbook of Clinical Pharmacology and Therapeutics*,
b) True   Chapter 34. Prophylactic broad-spectrum intravenous
c) True   antibiotics are commonly used, especially if there is
d) True   evidence of infection (e.g. spontaneous peritonitis).
e) True   Intravenous acetylcysteine is also used but its precise
value is yet to be fully confirmed

276 a) True   See *Textbook of Clinical Pharmacology and Therapeutics*,
b) False   Chapter 34. Terlipressin is a derivative of vasopressin
c) False   (antidiuretic hormone). Octreotide is an analogue of
d) True   somatostatin
e) False

277 a) False   – Usually mild and asymptomatic increase in transaminases
b) False   – Hepatic fibrosis/cirrhosis
c) True   – Rare now that low-dose oestrogens are more commonly
prescribed
d) True   – Associated with fever, abdominal pain and pruritus
e) True   – Usually transient

278 a) True   – A lipase inhibitor. Adverse effects include rectal leakage
and oily faeces
b) True   – Sibutramine inhibits the reuptake of noradrenaline and
serotonin. It is not licensed for use for longer than 1 year
c) False   – Transient weight loss secondary to fluid loss
d) False   – Inhibits $5HT_2$ receptors, increases appetite and causes
weight gain
e) False   – Although dexamphetamine decreases appetite, it has
considerable abuse potential. This and adverse effects
which include insomnia, restlessness, convulsions,
tachycardia, hypertension severely limits its use to
specialist treatment of narcolepsy and attention deficit
disorder

279 a) False   Rimonabant is an oral, selective, cannabinoid CB1 receptor
b) False   antagonist which is used as an adjunct to diet to achieve
c) False   weight loss. It is not licensed for use for longer than 2 years
d) True
e) True

EMQ ANSWERS

280 ALIMENTARY SYSTEM

1 F Ondansetron is a $5HT_3$ antagonist which is very effective in the prevention and treatment of acute nausea and vomiting secondary to cytotoxic chemotherapy and radiotherapy as well as following abdominal surgery.

2 E Loperamide is an effective, well-tolerated antidiarrhoeal agent. It is an opioid that does not, under normal circumstances, cross the blood–brain barrier.

3 G Olsalazine is a prodrug consisting of a dimer of two 5-aminosalicylic acid (5ASA) molecules linked by an azo bond. The azo bond is cleaved by colonic bacteria liberating 5ASA to the colon. In common with other aminosalicylates, olsalazine helps maintain remission in ulcerative colitis.

4 A Gemcitabine is an option for first-line chemotherapy for patients with advanced or metastatic adenocarcinoma of the pancreas.

5 J Ribavarin and peginterferon alfa are used in combination to treat chronic hepatitis C.

CHAPTER SEVEN

ENDOCRINE SYSTEM

MULTIPLE CHOICE QUESTIONS

281 In young, insulin-dependent diabetic (type 1 diabetic) patients:

a) There is good evidence that improved diabetic control reduces the incidence of microvascular complications
b) Blood glucose monitoring should be performed at home
c) Inhaled insulin should be tried before subcutaneous insulin
d) The dietary carbohydrate content should be 45–55 per cent of total calories
e) A fibre-rich diet reduces peak plasma glucose after meals and reduces insulin requirements

282 Recombinant human insulin in diabetes mellitus:

a) Never produces allergic reactions
b) The effective dose may be less than animal insulin
c) Patients are less aware of hypoglycaemia
d) Should not be given intravenously
e) Is not of any value in type 2 diabetes mellitus

283 A 17-year-old woman is admitted comatose with diabetic ketoacidosis. The following is accepted as 'standard of care':

a) Administer 500 mL of 0.9 per cent saline in the first 2 hours
b) Bladder catheterization
c) Administer subcutaneous insulin 0.1 unit/kg/hour
d) Administer 8.4 per cent sodium bicarbonate intravenously if the arterial pH is between 7.2 and 7.3
e) Aspiration of the stomach

284 Sulphonylureas:

a) Are used in obese diabetics who show a tendency to ketosis
b) Improve symptoms of polyuria and polydipsia
c) Have been proven to reduce the vascular complications of type 2 diabetics
d) Require functioning beta cells for a hypoglycaemic effect
e) Are usually administered once daily at bed time

285 Gliclazide:

a) Should never be combined with acarbose
b) Can be safely prescribed concomitantly with an angiotensin-converting enzyme (ACE) inhibitor
c) Hypoglycaemia can be reversed by intramuscular glucagon
d) Should not be prescribed concurrently with metformin
e) Stimulates appetite

286 Metformin, a biguanide:

a) May cause lactic acidosis
b) Is particularly useful in alcoholic diabetic patients
c) Causes hypoglycaemia in non-diabetic patients
d) Should be discontinued before major elective surgery
e) Causes anorexia and weight loss

287 'Glitazones' (e.g. pioglitazone and rosiglitazone):

a) Are indicated in type 1 diabetes
b) Bind to peroxisome proliferating activator receptor γ (PPAR γ), a nuclear receptor found mainly in adipocytes and also in hepatocytes and myocytes
c) Have a rapid onset of action and should be taken shortly before each main meal
d) Reduce peripheral insulin resistance
e) Are associated with weight gain and fluid retention

288 Carbimazole:

a) Decreases thyroid hormone synthesis
b) Inhibits the peripheral conversion of T_4 to the more active T_3
c) Should be stopped immediately if a rash develops
d) Has an active metabolite
e) Is associated with neutropenia

289 In a thyroid crisis with hyperpyrexia, tachycardia, vomiting, dehydration and shock the following are usually indicated:

a) Metaraminol
b) Propranolol
c) Intravenous saline
d) Glucocorticoids
e) Aspirin

290 The following may cause hypercalcaemia:
  a) Cinacalcet
  b) Calcitonin
  c) Bisphosphonates
  d) Alfacalcidol (1α-hydroxycholecalciferol)
  e) Thiazide diuretics

291 Disodium etidronate is used:
  a) Orally because it has high oral bioavailability
  b) In Paget's disease
  c) In hypercalcaemia of malignancy
  d) With calcium carbonate in established vertebral osteoporosis
  e) To inhibit bone resorption and formation

292 Glucocorticoids:
  a) Reduce circulating numbers of eosinophils by inducing apoptosis
  b) Reduce circulating numbers of T lymphocytes
  c) Increase circulating numbers of neutrophils
  d) Increase circulating numbers of platelets
  e) Increase the transcription of proteins such as tumour necrosis factor (TNF), interleukin 1 (IL-1) and granulocyte colony-stimulating factor (G-CSF)

293 Rapid withdrawal after prolonged prednisolone administration can cause:
  a) Acute adrenal insufficiency
  b) Malaise
  c) Hypercalciuria
  d) Arthralgia
  e) Fever

294 Chronic administration of corticosteroids (iatrogenic Cushing's syndrome) results in:
  a) Increased susceptibility to opportunistic infection
  b) Hyperkalaemia
  c) Hypertension
  d) Posterior capsular cataracts
  e) Proximal myopathy

295 Oral corticosteroid (e.g. prednisolone) therapy is indicated in:
  a) Fibrosing alveolitis
  b) Temporal arteritis
  c) Viral meningitis
  d) Diabetes insipidus
  e) Idiopathic thrombocytopenic purpura

296 The risk of thromboembolic disease associated with use of the combined oral contraceptive is increased in women:
a) Over 35 years of age
b) Who smoke
c) Who have been using oral contraceptives continuously for 5 years or more
d) Who take St John's wort
e) Who have known protein C or protein S deficiency

297 Adverse effects associated with the combined oral contraceptive include:
a) Aggravation of asthma
b) Stroke in women with migraine
c) Nephrotic syndrome
d) Peripheral neuropathy
e) Budd–Chiari syndrome

298 The following are indications to stop the oral contraceptive immediately (pending investigation and treatment):
a) Haemoptysis
b) Jaundice
c) Concurrent rifabutin therapy
d) First (unexplained) epileptic seizure
e) Severe unilateral calf pain

299 Post-coital contraception consisting of levonorgestrol given within 72 hours of unprotected intercourse:
a) Has a failure rate of less than 10 per cent
b) Is less effective than having a copper intrauterine device (IUD) inserted within 5 days of unprotected sexual intercourse
c) If vomiting occurs within 3 hours of ingestion, that dose should be repeated
d) Asthma is a contraindication
e) The next menstrual bleed may be early or late

300 Bromocriptine:
a) Stimulates lactation
b) Is used to treat hyperprolactinaemia
c) Is a dopamine D_2 receptor agonist
d) Commonly causes diarrhoea
e) Is effective in reducing symptoms of the syndrome of inappropriate antidiuretic hormone (ADH) secretion

301 There is reliable evidence that giving oestrogen for several years starting at the menopause to a woman with an intact uterus:
a) Reduces risk of osteoporosis
b) Reduces risk of coronary artery disease
c) Reduces age-related decline in cognitive function
d) Increases risk of stroke
e) Increases risk of breast cancer

302 Octreotide:
a) Is a synthetic peptide with a molecular weight of 10 000
b) Is effective in reducing symptoms of carcinoid syndrome
c) Is effective in treating diarrhoea states induced by irinotecan cancer chemotherapy
d) Commonly causes hyperglycaemia
e) Is effective in the acute treatment of bleeding from oesophageal varices

303 Clomifene:
a) Is an oestrogen receptor agonist
b) Is used in infertility treatment
c) Reduces follicle-stimulating hormone/luteinizing hormone (FSH/LH) secretion
d) Causes multiple births
e) Can cause acute psychotic reactions

304 The following may help alleviate symptoms associated with prostatic hyperplasia:
a) Clonidine
b) Tamsulosin
c) Doxazosin
d) Cyproterone acetate
e) Finasteride

305 Sildenafil:
a) Is administered by intracavernosal injection
b) Inhibits prostaglandin E_1
c) Inhibits type V phosphodiesterase
d) Potentiates the action of organic nitrates
e) May cause headaches, flushing, nasal congestion and disturbances of colour vision

Answers: see pages 129–132

EXTENDED MATCHING QUESTIONS

306 DIABETES MELLITUS

A	Bendroflumethiazide		F	Gliclazide
B	Inhaled insulin		G	Pioglitazone
C	Glucagon		H	Orlistat
D	Insulin glargine		I	Insulin lispro
E	Acarbose		J	Metformin

Link each of 1 to 5 below with the most appropriate item from A to J:

1   Lactic acidosis
2   Rapid hypoglycaemic effect
3   Useful in treatment of hypoglycaemia in a comatose patient
4   Action on a nuclear receptor
5   Depolarizes pancreatic islet beta cells

307 THYROID

A	Salbutamol		F	^{131}I
B	Carbimazole		G	Thyroxine
C	Lithium		H	Lugol's iodine
D	Imatinib		I	Thyrotropin-releasing hormone (TRH)
E	Tri-iodothyronine		J	Amiodarone

Link each of 1 to 5 below with the most appropriate item from A to J:

1   Rapid onset of thyroid action
2   Its principal metabolite inhibits peroxidase in the thyroid
3   Preparation for surgery on a toxic goitre
4   Treatment of thyroid carcinoma
5   Associated with goitre, hypo- or hyper-thyroidism

308 CALCIUM METABOLISM

A	Calcitonin		F	Calcium carbonate
B	Alfacalcidol		G	Zinc sulphate
C	Strontium ranelate		H	Calciferol
D	Cinacalcet		I	Teriparatide
E	Risedronate		J	Chlortalidone

Link each of 1 to 5 below with the most appropriate item from A to J:

1   Indicated in renal osteodystrophy
2   Phosphate-binding agent
3   Prevention and treatment of osteoporosis
4   Enhances signalling through the calcium-sensing receptor
5   May raise the serum calcium, glucose and urate whilst lowering the
    serum potassium

309 ADRENAL

A	Metyrapone	F	Aldosterone
B	Fludrocortisone	G	Isoprenaline
C	Dexamethasone	H	Phenoxybenzamine
D	Adrenaline	I	Dipivefrine
E	Aliskiren	J	Spironolactone

Link each of 1 to 5 below with the most appropriate item from A to J:

1 Helpful in controlling symptoms of Cushing's disease
2 Reduces cerebral oedema associated with brain tumour
3 Used therapeutically for its mineralocorticoid action
4 Irreversible alpha receptor antagonist
5 The main adrenal mineralocorticoid

310 PITUITARY

A	Octreotide	F	Demeclocycline
B	Atosiban	G	Pegvisomant
C	Goserelin	H	Tetracosactide
D	Somatropin	I	L-Arginine
E	Desmopressin	J	Prolactin

Link each of 1 to 5 below with the most appropriate item from A to J:

1 Long-acting somatostatin analogue
2 Downregulates FSH/LH release
3 Stimulation test to exclude Addison's disease
4 Growth hormone receptor antagonist
5 Treatment of syndrome of inappropriate antidiuretic hormone secretion (SIADH)

ANSWERS: see pages 133–134

MCQ ANSWERS

281 a) True   In insulin-dependent diabetes mellitus (IDDM), in addition
       b) True   to tight diabetic control which can usually be achieved by
       c) False   education and insulin two or three times daily plus diet,
       d) True   there must be regular screening for microvascular
       e) True   complications. Laser therapy of early proliferative
                       retinopathy prevents blindness

282 a) False   – But are much less common than with animal insulin
       b) True   – Possibly due to fewer blocking antibodies
       c) False   – Initial fears unfounded following double-blind studies
       d) False
       e) False   – If target glucose values in type 2 diabetes mellitus are not
                       achieved with diet and oral glucose-lowering-agents,
                       insulin is used

283 a) False   – 1.5–2 L over the first 2 hours
       b) True   – Helps in accurate monitoring of urine output. A central
                       venous pressure line also aids fluid management
       c) False   – Give intravenous short-acting insulin via syringe pump
       d) False   – May worsen intracellular and cerebrospinal acidaemia
       e) True   – Gastric stasis is common and inhalation of vomit can be
                       fatal. Insertion of a cuffed endotracheal tube may be
                       necessary before nasogastric aspiration depending on the
                       patient's level of consciousness

284 a) False
       b) True
       c) False   – Early and effective treatment of hypertension does reduce
                       the macro- and microvascular complications of diabetes
       d) True   – Increase plasma insulin concentrations
       e) False   – Most commonly as a single dose with breakfast

285 a) False   Acarbose is a reversible competitive inhibitor of intestinal
       b) True   alpha-glucoside hydrolases and delays the absorption of
                       starch and sucrose, but does not affect the absorption of
                       ingested glucose
       c) True   – A useful alternative to intravenous glucose if the patient is
                       unable to take glucose orally and venous access is
                       impractical (e.g. in the home) or unavailable
       d) False
       e) True   – cf. metformin

286 a) True   Metformin is particularly useful in obese patients with
    b) False   non-insulin-dependent (type 2) diabetes mellitus
    c) False   uncontrolled by diet and a sulphonylurea.
    d) True   Lactic acidosis is the most sinister adverse effect and
    e) True   has a high mortality. Metformin is contraindicated in
                     renal/hepatic/cardiac failure because of the increased
                     risk of lactic acidosis

287 a) False   The 'glitazones' reduce peripheral insulin resistance
    b) True   leading to a reduction in blood glucose concentration.
    c) False   Whilst use of 'glitazones' lowers HbA_{1c} (glycated
    d) True   haemoglobin) in type 2 diabetes mellitus patients
    e) True   inadequately controlled on diet $\pm$ other oral
                     hypoglycaemic drugs, an effect on mortality or diabetic
                     complications is currently unproven. There is a possible
                     increased risk of cardiac failure associated with 'glitazones'
                     in diabetic patients

288 a) True
    b) False   – In contrast to propylthiouracil and beta blockers
    c) False   – Pruritus and rashes are common. They may be treated with
                      antihistamines or propylthiouracil substituted for the
                      carbimazole if symptoms are significant
    d) True   – Methimazole, which is responsible for the therapeutic action
    e) True   – Potentially life-threatening/fatal

289 a) False   A thyroid crisis requires emergency treatment with
    b) True   intravenous fluids, propranolol, hydrocortisone, oral
    c) True   iodine and propylthiouracil or carbimazole
    d) True
    e) False

290 a) False   Hypercalcaemia may be a life-threatening emergency.
    b) False   General management includes rehydration and
    c) False   maintenance of hydration with physiological saline.
    d) True   Cinacalcet sensitizes calcium-sensing receptors and is used
    e) True   in secondary hyperparathyroidism. Calcitonin and
                      bisphosphonates reduce the plasma calcium.
                      Glucocorticoids reduce plasma calcium in sarcoidosis

291 a) False   Is given intravenously or orally in spite of poor systemic
    b) True   bioavailability (1–5 per cent). It is generally well tolerated
    c) True
    d) True
    e) True

292 a) True   Glucocorticoids reduce transcription of many
    b) True   proinflammatory genes and induce the transcription of
    c) True   others, e.g. lipocortin which inhibits phospholipase

d) True   A$_2$ and consequently inhibits the formation of several proinflammatory mediators. The anti-inflammatory action takes 6–8 hours to manifest after dosing

e) False   – Glucocorticosteroids inhibit the transcription of proinflammatory cytokines such as TNF, IL-1, etc.

293 a) True   Even in patients who have been successfully weaned from
b) True   chronic steroid therapy, an acute stress (e.g. trauma,
c) False   surgery, infection) may precipitate an acute adrenal crisis
d) True
e) True

294 a) True   – For example fungal infections and tuberculosis – may reactivate old tuberculous lesions
b) False   – Hypokalaemia (aldosterone-like effect)
c) True
d) True   – In addition local application of steroids to the eye predisposes to infection
e) True

295 a) True   – Not curative but delays deterioriation in some patients
b) True   – May prevent irreversible loss of vision
c) False
d) False
e) True

296 a) True   The combined oral contraceptive should be stopped four
b) True   weeks before major elective surgery
c) True
d) False   – St John's wort is likely to induce metabolism of steroids, reducing their efficacy and side-effect risks
e) True   – Such patients have a high risk of thromboembolism because the lack of these proteins produces a procoagulable state

297 a) False   The overall acceptability of the combined pill is 80 per cent;
b) True   minor side-effects can often be controlled by a change in
c) False   preparation
d) False
e) True

298 a) True   Other indications to stop the combined oral contraceptive
b) True   immediately include sudden severe chest pain, sudden
c) False   unilateral calf pain, serious neurological effects, hepatitis,
d) True   hepatomegaly, severe depression and hypertension
e) True

299 a) True   Urgent medical attention is necessary if lower abdominal
b) True   pain occurs, as it could signify an ectopic pregnancy.
c) True   Mifepristone, a progesterone antagonist, is an unlicensed
d) False   alternative post-coital contraceptive
e) True

300 a) False – Suppresses lactation
b) True
c) True
d) False – The commonest adverse effects are nausea and constipation and orthostatic hypotension
e) False – Fluid restriction and demeclocycline is usually effective

301 a) True   Hormone replacement therapy (HRT) using small doses of
b) False   oestrogen (with progesterone if uterus intact) alleviates
c) False   menopausal symptoms such as vaginal atrophy and
d) True   vasomotor instability
e) True

302 a) False – It is a synthetic octapeptide of eight amino acids, molecular weight approx. 900
b) True
c) True
d) True – It antagonizes insulin release
e) True

303 a) False – It is an anti-oestrogen
b) True
c) False – It blocks oestrogen receptors in the hypothalamus, feedback inhibition of FSH/LH is reduced and FSH/LH secretion increases
d) True
e) True

304 a) False – A central alpha$_2$ and imidazoline agonist that is useful for menopausal vasomotor symptoms
b) True – Selective alpha blocker
c) True – Selective alpha blocker
d) False – An anti-androgen used in the treatment of severe hypersexuality and sexual deviation in the male. It may be used as an adjunct in inoperable prostate cancer
e) True – Finasteride inhibits 5α-reductase, reducing prostate size. Adverse effects include decreased libido and impotence

305 a) False   Sildenafil, a phosphodiesterase type 5 inhibitor, is used for
b) False   the treatment of erectile dysfunction. It is taken by mouth
c) True   approximately 1 hour before sexual activity. Concomitant
d) True   nitrates are contraindicated
e) True

306 DIABETES MELLITUS

1 **J** Metformin is the drug of choice in overweight diabetic patients in whom diet is inadequate. It should be avoided in patients with renal impairment due to the risk of lactic acidosis.

2 **I** Insulin lispro has a more rapid and shorter duration of hypoglycaemic action than natural insulin.

3 **C** Glucagon, via stimulation of adenyl cyclase, stimulates glycogen breakdown and gluconeogenesis.

4 **G** Pioglitazone binds to PPAR γ, a nuclear receptor.

5 **F** Gliclazide, a sulphonylurea, depolarizes pancreatic islet beta cells, thereby stimulating insulin secretion.

307 THYROID

1 **E** Tri-iodothyronine (T_3) is more potent and has a more rapid onset of action than thyroxine (T_4).

2 **B** Methimazole, the principal metabolite of carbimazole, inhibits peroxidase in the thyroid. Granulocytopenia is a severe adverse drug effect.

3 **H** Lugol's iodine is useful for suppressing thyroid activity prior to the thyroidectome.

4 **F** ^{131}I is used to treat thyrotoxicosis (from Graves' disease or toxic nodular goitre) and is also used in high dose for thyroid carcinoma as it can be taken up by metastases and thus deliver radiotherapy locally to the tumour.

5 **J** Several drugs cause goitre, including lithium and imatinib, but amiodarone is unusual in being associated not only with goitre but also with either underactive or overactive thyroid.

308 CALCIUM METABOLISM

1 **B** Calciferol (regular vitamin D) is not effective in patients with renal failure because it needs to be hydroxylated in the kidney. Such patients require preparations such as alfacalcidol or calcitriol.

2 **F** Calcium carbonate and aluminium hydroxide are used as phosphate-binding agents in the management of hyperphosphataemia in renal failure.

3 **E** Risedronate and other bisphosphonates are used for the prevention and treatment of osteoporosis.

4 D Cinacalcet enhances signalling through the calcium-sensing receptor reducing parathyroid hormone. It is licensed for the treatment of secondary hyperparathyroidism in dialysis patients with renal failure and in parathyroid carcinoma to reduce serum calcium concentration.

5 J Chlortalidone and the related thiazide diuretics are associated with the following metabolic consequences: hypokalaemia, hypomagnesaemia, hyponatraemia, hypercalcaemia, hypochloraemic alkalosis, hyperuricaemia and hyperglycaemia.

309 ADRENAL

1 A Metyrapone is a competitive inhibitor of 11β-hydroxylation in the adrenal cortex.

2 C Dexamethasone is used relatively short term (as a diagnostic test, or to treat cerebral oedema).

3 B Fludrocortisone may be combined with hydrocortisone since hydrocortisone alone may not possess sufficient mineralocorticoid activity for complete replacement in patients with adrenal insufficiency.

4 H Phenoxybenzamine is an irreversible alpha-receptor antagonist indicated in hypertensive episodes in phaeochromocytoma, and to prepare patients with phaeochromocytoma for surgery.

5 F Aldosterone has no glucocorticoid activity, but is 1000 times more active than hydrocortisone as a mineralocorticoid. Its effects can be blocked by spironolactone.

310 PITUITARY

1 A Octreotide is a long-acting somatostatin analogue used for the relief of symptoms related to neuroendocrine (particularly carcinoid) tumours and acromegaly. It is also used (unlicensed) in the management of variceal bleeding.

2 C Goserelin is an analogue of gonadotrophin-releasing hormone. It initially stimulates the release of FSH/LH, but then downregulates this response (usually after two weeks) effectively leading to medical orchidectomy/ovariectomy.

3 H Tetracosactide is a synthetic analogue of adrenocorticotrophic hormone (ACTH).

4 G Pegvisomant is a genetically modified analogue of human growth hormone, which acts as an antagonist to growth hormone.

5 F First-line treatment of SIADH is to restrict fluid intake. Demeclocycline blocks ADH action on the kidney and may be used in addition.

CHAPTER EIGHT

SELECTIVE TOXICITY

MULTIPLE CHOICE QUESTIONS

311 The following antibacterial drugs inhibit folic acid biosynthesis:
 a) Amoxicillin
 b) Aztreonam
 c) Levofloxacin
 d) Trimethoprim
 e) Sulfonamides

312 The following infections have been paired with appropriate antibacterial therapy:
 a) Acute otitis media – amoxicillin
 b) Acute epiglottitis in children – cefotaxime/ceftriaxone or chloramphenicol
 c) Legionnaire's disease – erythromycin and rifampicin
 d) Acute cystitis arising outside hospital in adults – trimethoprim
 e) Antibiotic-associated pseudomembranous colitis – oral vancomycin

313 The following antibacterial drug combinations are of accepted benefit in the treatment of the stated infection:
 a) Amoxicillin and cefadroxil for lower urinary tract infection in severely ill patients
 b) Phenoxymethylpenicillin and tetracycline for acute osteomyelitis in a child under 5 years
 c) Isoniazid, rifampicin, pyrazinamide and ethambutol in the initial treatment for pulmonary tuberculosis (TB)
 d) Erythromycin and tetracycline for septicaemia
 e) Metronidazole and nitrofurantoin for non-specific urethritis

314 The following anti-infective drugs are suitable as prophylaxis in the stated conditions:
- **a)** Co-amoxiclav – human and animal bites
- **b)** Ciprofloxacin – close adult contacts of meningococcal disease
- **c)** Flucloxacillin – prevention of a secondary case of diphtheria
- **d)** Erythromycin – whooping cough contact in an unvaccinated child under 1 year old
- **e)** Aciclovir – close contacts of patients with herpes labialis

315 Benzylpenicillin:
- **a)** Is inactivated in gastric acid
- **b)** Is effective in meningococcal infections
- **c)** Has a half-life of 24 hours
- **d)** Is less susceptible than flucloxacillin to beta-lactamase-producing strains of staphylococci
- **e)** Approximately 1 in 500 injections cause anaphylactic shock

316 Amoxicillin:
- **a)** Unlike benzylpenicillin is not susceptible to beta-lactamases
- **b)** Is effective against many strains of *Haemophilus influenzae*
- **c)** Is ineffective in most cases of community-acquired urinary tract infections
- **d)** Drug-related skin rashes may appear after dosing has stopped
- **e)** Drug-related skin rashes are more common in patients with infectious mononucleosis

317 The following drugs are effective in staphylococcal infections:
- **a)** Ampicillin
- **b)** Co-amoxiclav
- **c)** Fusidic acid
- **d)** Flucloxacillin
- **e)** Metronidazole

318 Cefuroxime:
- **a)** Has activity against streptococci
- **b)** Has no activity against Gram-negative organisms
- **c)** Plasma concentrations should be monitored to avoid toxicity
- **d)** Is principally renally eliminated
- **e)** Has approximately 5–10 per cent cross-sensitivity for allergic reactions with benzylpenicillin

319 Gentamicin, an aminoglycoside:
 a) Is effective in pneumococcal pneumonia
 b) Is poorly absorbed from the gut
 c) Has an elimination half-life of approximately 12 hours if renal function is normal
 d) Cerebrospinal fluid (CSF) penetration is poor
 e) Causes irreversible eighth nerve damage

320 Chloramphenicol is usually effective in:
 a) Pulmonary tuberculosis
 b) Epiglottitis
 c) Typhoid
 d) Bacterial meningitis
 e) Bacterial conjunctivitis

321 Uses of clarithromycin include:
 a) *Mycoplasma pneumoniae*
 b) Legionnaire's disease
 c) *Campylobacter* enteritis
 d) Non-specific urethritis
 e) Meningococcal meningitis

322 Erythromycin:
 a) Is poorly absorbed when given by mouth
 b) Has a shorter half-life than azithromycin
 c) The most common adverse effect is headache
 d) Inhibits CYP450 enzymes
 e) Cannot be prescribed with amoxicillin

323 Tetracyclines are used to treat:
 a) Infections caused by *Clostridium difficile*
 b) Lyme disease
 c) Acne vulgaris
 d) Systemic lupus erythematosus
 e) Non-specific urethritis

324 Metronidazole is used to treat:
 a) Trichomonal infections
 b) Amoebic dysentry
 c) Giardiasis
 d) Tetanus
 e) Gas gangrene

325 Ciprofloxacin:

a) Is a drug of first choice in *Streptococcus pneumoniae* infections
b) Is effective in *Pseudomonas* infections
c) Should be avoided in children
d) Should be avoided in epileptics
e) Is ineffective if administered orally

326 Isoniazid:

a) Undergoes acetylation (by *N*-acetyltransferase) in the liver
b) Is used for only the initial two months of the recommended six-month anti-TB regimen in the UK
c) Is readily absorbed from the gut
d) Does not diffuse into the CSF
e) Is contraindicated in children under the age of 10 years

327 Adverse effects associated with rifampicin include:

a) Hepatitis and cholestatic jaundice
b) Peripheral neuropathy
c) Convulsions
d) Influenza-like symptoms
e) Pink/red urine and tears

328 Rifampicin accelerates the CYP450-mediated metabolism of:

a) Corticosteroids
b) Warfarin
c) Streptomycin
d) Digoxin
e) Oestrogen

329 The following adverse effects are correctly paired with a causative antituberculous drug:

a) Peripheral neuropathy – isoniazid
b) Ototoxicity – rifampicin
c) Hyperuricaemia – pyrazinamide
d) Retrobulbar neuritis – ethambutol
e) Hepatotoxicity – streptomycin

330 Dapsone:

a) Is used in the treatment of amoebiasis
b) Is indicated in multibacillary leprosy
c) Is used in the treatment of dermatitis herpetiformis
d) Is acetylated in the liver
e) Has cross-sensitivity with sulfonamides

331 Amphotericin:
a) Is effective in local *Candida* spp. infections
b) Is effective in systemic *Candida* spp. infections
c) Is nephrotoxic
d) Causes hypokalaemia
e) Is ineffective in cryptococcosis

332 The following antifungal agents have been paired correctly with an appropriate indication:
a) Nystatin – oral *Candida* infections
b) Voriconazole – invasive aspergillosis
c) Flucytosine – tinea pedis
d) Clotrimazole – intertrigo
e) Miconazole – cold sores

333 Voriconazole:
a) Is available and effective as oral and intravenous therapy
b) Is active against *Aspergillus*
c) Inhibits cortisol biosynthesis
d) Inhibits CYP3A
e) Gastrointestinal absorption is reduced by omeprazole

334 Fluconazole:
a) Oral absorption is minimal unless taken on an empty stomach
b) Presystemic metabolism is extensive
c) Penetrates the central nervous system well
d) Is excreted 80 per cent by the kidney
e) Causes gynaecomastia

335 Terbinafine:
a) Is indicated in dermatophyte nail infections
b) A topical preparation is indicated in ringworm infection (e.g. tinea pedis/cruris)
c) A single dose is usually effective
d) Is a potent CYP450 enzyme inducer
e) May exacerbate psoriasis

336 Aciclovir:
a) Inhibits viral DNA polymerase
b) Is indicated in herpetic keratitis
c) Should be avoided if possible in pregnancy
d) Is indicated in herpetic meningoencephalitis
e) Is ineffective in chicken pox

337 Foscarnet:

a) Is indicated in cytomegalovirus (CMV) retinitis in acquired immune deficiency syndrome (AIDS) patients
b) Aciclovir-resistant herpes simplex virus infections
c) Is nephrotoxic
d) Causes fits
e) Is usually administered by mouth or topically

338 Ribavarin:

a) Is indicated in CMV retinitis in AIDS patients
b) Inhibits viral RNA methyltransferase
c) Must be taken up into cells and phosphorylated to be effective
d) Can be administered via aerosol inhalation to treat bronchiolitis
e) Is combined with interferon alfa in the treatment of hepatitis C

339 The following are used in the prophylaxis or treatment of influenza:

a) Amantadine
b) Palivizumab
c) Entecavir
d) Oseltamivir
e) Zanamivir

340 Adverse effects associated with the interferons include:

a) Hypocalcaemia
b) Inhibition of spermatogenesis
c) Renal tubular acidosis
d) Lymphopenia
e) Influenza-like symptoms

341 One or more of the interferons are indicated in:

a) Herpes simplex encephalitis
b) Chronic hepatitis B infection
c) Chronic hepatitis C infection
d) Hairy cell leukaemia
e) CMV retinitis

342 Which of the following antiretroviral drug combinations is accepted first-line therapy for patients with human immunodeficiency virus (HIV) infection?

a) Zidovudine (AZT) plus 2,3-dideoxycytidine (ddC)
b) AZT + lamivudine + lopinavir/ritonavir
c) Ritonavir + amprenavir + enfuvirtide
d) AZT + lamivudine + nevirapine
e) AZT + stavudine (d4T) + enfuvirtide

343 Properties of HIV protease inhibitors include:
  a) Cause hypertriglyceridaemia and truncal fat redistribution
  b) Are most effective of the antiretrovirals at reducing plasma HIV RNA copy number
  c) Oral bioavailability is consistent and >95 per cent
  d) Cause many drug–drug interactions due to inhibition of CYP3A
  e) HIV resistance to one agent in the class usually means cross-resistance to others

344 The following are used to treat *Pneumocystis carinii* pneumonia (PCP) in patients with HIV infection:
  a) Aztreonam
  b) Intravenous co-trimoxazole
  c) Rifabutin
  d) Pentamidine
  e) Glucocorticosteroids if the arterial Po_2 is less than 60 mmHg

345 Quinine sulfate:
  a) Is the drug of choice in chloroquine-resistant falciparum malaria
  b) Is available for intravenous and oral use
  c) Is effective in eradicating the hepatic parasites in *Plasmodium vivax* malaria
  d) Is contraindicated in renal failure
  e) Large therapeutic doses cause tinnitus

346 The following adverse effects are paired with the correct causative antimalarial drug:
  a) Acneiform eruption – chloroquine
  b) Stevens–Johnson syndrome – quinine
  c) Psychosis – mefloquine
  d) Prolongation of QTc – proguanil
  e) Haemolytic anaemia – primaquine

347 The following infections have been paired with appropriate drug therapy:
  a) *Trypanosoma gambiense* (African sleeping sickness), early stages – pentamidine and suramin
  b) *Giardia lamblia* – metronidazole
  c) *Taenia saginata* (a tapeworm) – emetine
  d) *Strongyloides stercoralis* (threadworm) – mebendazole
  e) *Toxocara canis* – pyraquantal

348 The following anticancer drugs are considered highly emetogenic:
- **a)** Cyclophosphamide
- **b)** Methotrexate
- **c)** 5-Fluorouracil
- **d)** Interleukin 2
- **e)** Cisplatin

349 The following cytotoxic drugs may be associated with profound and prolonged myelosuppression:
- **a)** Chlorambucil
- **b)** Melphalan
- **c)** 1,3-bis (2 chloroethyl)-1-nitroso-urea (BCNU)
- **d)** Bleomycin
- **e)** Vincristine

350 During cancer chemotherapy:
- **a)** Infection is the commonest life-threatening complication
- **b)** Infection is often acquired from the patient's own gut flora
- **c)** If infection occurs, pyrexia is usually absent
- **d)** Men and women must be strongly advised to avoid conception
- **e)** There is a danger of inducing second malignancies

351 Cyclophosphamide:
- **a)** Is normally used in combination with other cytotoxic agents
- **b)** Is an alkylating agent
- **c)** Causes granulocytopenia
- **d)** Causes nausea and vomiting
- **e)** Causes alopecia

352 Methotrexate:
- **a)** Inhibits dihydrofolate reductase which synthesises tetrahydrofolate from dihydrofolate
- **b)** The toxicity of high doses can be reduced by giving folinic acid 24 hours after the methotrexate
- **c)** Is primarily excreted in the bile
- **d)** Chronic treatment can cause cirrhosis
- **e)** Is the first-line treatment for choriocarcinoma

353 The following cytotoxic drugs are paired with a characteristic adverse effect:
- **a)** Etoposide – peripheral neuropathy
- **b)** Paclitaxel – alopecia
- **c)** Daunorubicin – cardiomyopathy
- **d)** Irinotecan – diarrhoea
- **e)** 6-Mercaptopurine – pulmonary fibrosis

354 During cisplatin therapy:
   a) Pretreatment hydration is mandatory
   b) Pretreatment with dexamethasone and a $5HT_3$ antagonist (e.g. ondansetron) reduces the nausea and vomiting
   c) Visual disturbances are common
   d) Magnesium supplements are usually given
   e) Nephrotoxicity is dose related and dose limiting

355 Paclitaxel (a taxane):
   a) May be used alone or in combination for a broad range of epitheloid tumours and lymphomas
   b) Inhibits purine synthesis
   c) Causes sensory neuropathies
   d) Requires glucocorticosteroid premedication to minimize acute hypersensitivity reactions
   e) Is not associated with myelosuppression

356 Recombinant human erythropoietin is used to treat:
   a) Iron-deficient anaemia when iron is malabsorbed
   b) Sickle cell anaemia
   c) Anaemia of chronic renal failure
   d) AZT-related anaemia
   e) Clozapine-induced agranulocytosis

357 Filgrastim (human granulocyte colony-stimulating factor):
   a) Is usually administered by subcutaneous injection
   b) Causes immediate transient neutropenia
   c) Is used in myeloid leukaemia
   d) Stimulates proliferation and differentiation of myeloid progenitor cells
   e) Causes bone pain

358 Lopinavir, an HIV-protease inhibitor, is associated with the following:
   a) Lipodystrophy syndrome
   b) Hyperglycaemia
   c) Peripheral neuropathy
   d) Lactic acidosis
   e) Inhibition of metabolism of rifabutin

Answers: see pages 147–154

EXTENDED MATCHING QUESTIONS

359 ANTIBACTERIAL DRUGS

A	Oral vancomycin	F	Rifampicin
B	Trimethoprim	G	Ciprofloxacin
C	Flucloxacillin + fusidic acid	H	Gentamicin + metronidazole
D	Clarithromycin	I	Neomycin
E	Doxycycline	J	Amoxicillin

Which antibacterial drug or drug combination from the list above is the most appropriate choice for the infection scenarios listed below?

1   Lyme disease
2   Invasive salmonellosis
3   Antibiotic-associated colitis (pseudomembranous colitis)
4   Peritonitis in a patient allergic to cephalosporins
5   Uncomplicated community-acquired pneumonia in a penicillin-allergic patient

360 ANTIBACTERIAL DRUGS

A	Cefuroxime and clarithromycin	F	Ciprofloxacin
B	Benzylpenicillin and flucloxacillin	G	Erythromycin and rifampicin
C	Benzylpenicillin and gentamicin	H	Flucloxacillin and sodium fusidate
D	Ceftriaxone	I	Teicoplanin
E	Cefuroxime and metronidazole	J	Trimethoprim

From the above list, choose the most appropriate antibiotic regime for each of the following clinical situations:

1   A 35-year-old man severely ill with community-acquired pneumonia
2   A 40-year-old man with acute septic arthritis in his knee caused by *Staphylococcus aureus*
3   A 25-year-old woman with suspected bacterial meningitis
4   Suspected bacterial endocarditis following dental extraction in a 65-year-old man with mitral valve prolapse
5   A 38-year-old woman allergic to beta-lactam antibiotics with pyelonephritis

361 HIV

A	Azatanavir	F	Enfuvirtide
B	Rimantidine	G	Raltegravir
C	Efavirenz	H	Adefovir
D	Zidovudine (ZDV)	I	Ganciclovir
E	Zanamivir	J	Foscarnet

Match the correct drug with its pharmacodynamic effect (either on the HIV virus or the human host)

1   Competitive inhibition of the HIV reverse transcriptase
2   Inhibition of HIV entry into T cells
3   Non-competitive inhibition of HIV reverse transcriptase
4   Inhibition of HIV protease
5   Competitive inhibition of HIV integrase

362 HIV

A	Lopinavir	F	Maraviroc
B	Lamivudine	G	Abacavir
C	Nevirapine	H	Tenofovir
D	ZDV	I	Ganciclovir
E	Didanosine	J	Foscarnet

Match the drug with the correct property/side-effect defined below:

1   Active against HIV and CMV
2   Causes macrocytic anaemia with reticulocytopenia
3   Potent inhibitor of CYP3A and P-gp (ABCB1)
4   Does not require activation to a nucleotide
5   Oral bioavailability increased ('boosted') by ritonavir

363 MALARIA AND PARASITIC INFECTIONS

A	Atovaquone + proguanil	F	Mebendazole
B	Quinine	G	Diethylcarbamazine
C	Primaquine	H	Ivermectin
D	Artemesinin derivatives	I	Pentamidine
E	Niclosamide	J	Metronidazole

Select a drug/drug combination from the list above most appropriate for the indication below:

1   Acute falciparum malaria in a country with widespread chloroquine resistance (e.g. Ghana) where parenteral therapy is required
2   Malaria prophylaxis for a European tourist in Ghana
3   Eradication of hepatic forms of *P. vivax*
4   Threadworm infection in a 3-year-old child
5   Giardiasis

364 CANCER

A	Imatinib	F	Capecitabine
B	Oxaliplatin	G	Gemcitabine
C	Irinotecan	H	Gefitinib
D	Rituximab	I	Docetaxel
E	Trastuzumab	J	Bevacizumab

Match the drug with its correct molecular target:

1   BCR-Abl kinase
2   DNA Topoisomerase I
3   HER2/NEU (epidermal growth factor receptor-2 (EGFR-2))
4   Vascular endothelial growth factor (VEGF)
5   Epidermal growth factor receptor–tyrosine kinase (EGFR-TK)

365 CANCER

A	Dasatinib	F	Vincristine
B	Cisplatin	G	Doxorubicin
C	Fludarabine	H	Sorafenib
D	Interleukin 2	I	Paclitaxel
E	Interferon	J	Panimumomab

Match the drug with the correct common and serious adverse effect:

1   Hypothyroidism
2   Cerebellar ataxia
3   Acute renal tubular necrosis
4   Adult respiratory distress syndrome (non-cardiogenic pulmonary oedema)
5   Hypertension

ANSWERS: see pages 154–158

ANSWERS

MCQ ANSWERS

311 a) False   – Inhibits bacterial cell wall peptidoglycan cross-linking
     b) False   – Inhibits bacterial cell wall peptidoglycan cross-linking
     c) False   – Inhibit bacterial DNA gyrase (a bacterial DNA topoisomerase)
     d) True
     e) True

312 a) True   – When bacterial commonly caused by group A streptococci
     b) True   – Caused by *H. influenzae*
     c) True
     d) True
     e) True   – Caused by colonization of the colon with *Clostridium difficile*. Alternative oral metronidazole (NB: stop causative antibiotic)

313 a) False   – Intravenous gentamicin and cefuroxime
     b) False   – Caused commonly by *H. influenzae* or *Staphylococcus aureus* – amoxicillin and flucloxacillin is usually a satisfactory combination
     c) True   – Reduces the risk of TB resistance
     d) False   – Choice depends on clinical conditions, a beta-lactam and an aminoglycoside is a common bacteriocidal combination used for septicaemia
     e) False   – Single agent is effective (e.g. tetracycline or erythromycin)

314 a) True
     b) True
     c) False   – Erythromycin
     d) True
     e) False   – See *Textbook of Clinical Pharmacology and Therapeutics*, Chapters 43 and 45

315 a) True   – Whilst phenoxymethylpenicillin (penicillin V) is stable in gastric acid and is administered orally
     b) True
     c) False   – Short half-life of approximately 30 minutes
     d) False
     e) False   – 1 in 100 000

316 a) False   Amoxicillin is an extended-range penicillin used for chest
     b) True   infections, otitis media, urinary tract infection, biliary
     c) False   infections and prevention of bacterial endocarditis. Rashes
     d) True   are common and there is an especially high incidence in
     c) True   infectious mononucleosis and lymphatic leukaemia

317 a) False – Susceptible to beta-lactamases
b) True – A combination of amoxicillin with clavulanic acid (a beta-lactamase inhibitor)
c) True
d) True
e) False – Metronidazole is effective in anaerobic and protozoal infections. It is used as a part of triple therapy to eradicate *Helicobacter pylori*

318 a) True Cefuroxime combines lactamase stability with activity
b) False against streptococci, staphylococci, *H. influenzae* and
c) False *Escherichia coli*
d) True
e) True

319 a) False Aminoglycosides are used particularly in serious infections
b) True such as septicaemia, usually in combination with a beta-
c) False lactam (e.g. a penicillin). Blood concentration monitoring is
d) True mandatory to avoid toxicity. The half-life is approximately
e) True 2 hours if renal function is normal

320 a) False Chloramphenicol has a broad spectrum and penetrates
b) True tissues exceptionally well. Its widespread use in
c) True developing countries has led to some resistance. Its major
d) True disadvantage is a 1:40 000 incidence of aplastic anaemia
e) True (which can be irreversible)

321 a) True Macrolide antibiotics (erythromycin, clarithromycin and
b) True azithromycin), are useful alternatives to penicillin in
c) True penicillin-allergic patients (with the notable exception of
d) True meningitis) and are also effective against several unusual
e) False bacteria. Clarithromycin and azithromycin are given twice and once daily, respectively, unlike erythromycin which is given four times daily. They cause fewer gastrointestinal side-effects and show better tissue penetration (particularly azithromycin)

322 a) False – Well absorbed
b) True – Erythromycin, 1–1.5 hours; azithromycin, 40–60 hours
c) False – Gastrointestinal effects are most common
d) True – Causes accumulation of theophylline, warfarin and atorvastatin
e) False – They can be co-prescribed in e.g. community-acquired pneumonia

323 a) False Oral absorption of tetracyclines is reduced by food (except
b) True doxycycline). They must be avoided in renal impairment
c) True (except doxycycline)
d) False
e) True

324 a) True   Metronidazole has high activity against protozoa and
    b) True   anaerobic bacteria. It is widely used prophylactically before
    c) True   abdominal surgery when the rectal route is often suitable
    d) False
    e) True   – Often in conjunction with clindamycin

325 a) False   Oral bioavailability of the 4-fluoroquinolones is good and
    b) True   they offer an oral alternative to parenteral aminoglycosides
    c) True   and anti-pseudomonal penicillins for the treatment of
    d) True   pseudomonal infection. Quinolones cause arthropathy in
    e) False   young animals and can cause convulsions. Photosensitivity
                       also occurs

326 a) True   The recommended regimen for 'unsupervised treatment' of
                       pulmonary TB in the UK for a patient at low risk of poor
    b) False   compliance is isoniazid, rifampicin, ethambutol and
    c) True   pyrazinamide for two months followed by rifampicin and
    d) False   isoniazid for a further four months. Specialist advice
    e) False   should be sought for immunocompromised patients

327 a) True   Serious liver damage is uncommon but minor histological
    b) False   changes and rises in aminotransferase are common and in
    c) False   the absence of jaundice are not an indication for stopping
    d) True   treatment
    e) True

328 a) True   In women using the contraceptive pill, an alternative
    b) True   method of contraception should be provided. Streptomycin
    c) False   and digoxin are primarily cleared from the body by renal
    d) False   elimination
    e) True

329 a) True   – Use prophylactic pyridoxine in diabetics, alcoholics and the
                       malnourished – more common in slow acetylators
    b) False   – Occurs with streptomycin
    c) True   – May precipitate gout
    d) True   – Regular questioning for visual symptoms and baseline
                       assessment of visual acuity are essential. There must be
                       further visual examination if symptoms develop
    e) False   – Occurs with isoniazid, rifampicin and pyrazinamide

330 a) False   Dapsone is a sulfonamide derivative which is a competitive
    b) True   inhibitor of dihydropteroate (folate) synthetase, thereby
    c) True   inhibiting dihydrofolic acid production. Clofazimine
    d) True   and rifampicin are also used to treat leprosy
    e) True

331 a) True   Amphotericin is a broad-spectrum antifungal although
    b) True   *Aspergillus* spp. are usually resistant. It is administered
    c) True   topically (lozenges), orally (suspension) or intravenously.
    d) True   Thrombophlebitis is a common problem when used
    e) False   intravenously. Intravenous lipid formulations are less
                  nephrotoxic but more expensive

332 a) True   – NB: bitter taste
    b) True   – Alone or with flucytosine. Amphotericin is nephrotoxic
    c) False   – Used with amphotericin for systemic candidiasis and
                  cryptococcosis
    d) True   – Powder suitable
    e) False   – Cold sores are due to the virus herpes simplex

333 a) True
    b) True   – Voriconazole is a potent broad-spectrum triazole antifungal
                  active against *Candida* and *Aspergillus*
    c) True   – Inhibits enzymes involved in cortisol and testosterone
                  synthesis
    d) True   – Inhibits the metabolism of many drugs which are
                  metabolized by CYP3A
    e) False   – The absorption of fluconazole and voriconazole is not
                  significantly reduced by agents which increase gastric pH
                  (H_2 blockers or proton pump inhibitors)

334 a) False   Fluconazole is a potent and broad-spectrum antifungal
    b) False   drug. It may be used for local or systemic infections as well
    c) True   as prophylaxis in neutropenic patients. Adverse effects are
    d) True   gastrointestinal, erythema multiforme and hepatitis
    e) False

335 a) True   Terbinafine is available only as an oral preparation. It is
    b) False   used to treat ringworm or dermatophyte infections of the
    c) False   nails. It is usually given for 2–6 weeks (longer for nail bed
    d) False   infections)
    e) True

336 a) True   Aciclovir is a potent and selective inhibitor of herpes virus
    b) True   DNA polymerase. It may be administered as an ointment
    c) True   (e.g. in herpetic keratitis), orally (as in shingles) or by
    d) True   intravenous infusion as in encephalitis
    e) False

337 a) True   Foscarnet is a nucleotide analogue that inhibits viral DNA
    b) True   polymerase and thus DNA synthesis. It is administered as
    c) True   an intravenous infusion in both immunocompetent and

d) True   immunosuppressed patients
e) False

338 a) False   – Ganciclovir
     b) True   – NB: Ribavarin is a potent teratogen
     c) True
     d) True
     e) True

339 a) True   – Also used in Parkinson's disease
     b) False   – Monoclonal antibody used in prevention of respiratory
                    syncytial virus (RSV) infection in at-risk children
     c) False   – Entecavir is used to treat chronic hepatitis B infection
     d) True   – Oral administration
     e) True   – By inhalation only

340 a) False   – Associated with foscarnet
     b) False   – Associated with ganciclovir which is indicated in
                    severe CMV infection in immunocompromised patients
     c) False   – Associated with amphotericin
     d) True
     e) True

341 a) False   Interferons are glycoproteins secreted by cells infected
     b) True   with viruses or foreign double-stranded DNA. They are
     c) True   non-antigenic and species specific. Interferon alfa is
     d) True   combined with ribavirin for the treatment of hepatitis C.
     e) False   Interferon beta is licensed for the treatment of multiple
                    sclerosis

342 a) False   Triple therapy: two nucleoside reverse transcriptase inhibitors
     b) True   plus HIV protease inhibitor or plus a non-nucleoside reverse
     c) False   transcriptase inhibitor is accepted first-line therapy. See
     d) True   *Textbook of Clinical Pharmacology and Therapeutics*, Chapter 46
     e) False   – AZT + d4T antagonistic *in vitro* at least. Not used
                    clinically

343 a) True   Saquinavir, ritonavir, indinavir, lopinavir, amprenavir,
     b) True   atazanavir, tripanavir and nelfinavir are anti-HIV protease
     c) False   inhibitors
     d) True
     e) True

344 a) False   High-dose co-trimoxazole is first-line standard treatment
     b) True   for PCP in patients with HIV infection. After recovery,
     c) False   secondary prophylaxis with oral co-trimoxazole is usual.
     d) True   Rifabutin is indicated for prophylaxis of *Mycobacterium*
     e) True   *avium intracellulare* infections in HIV patients with low CD4
                    count

345 a) True – If resistance is not a possibility, chloroquine may be used
b) True
c) False – Primaquine
d) False
e) True – Cinchonism, which also includes deafness, headache, nausea and visual disturbance

346 a) True – Other choroquine side-effects include convulsions, visual disturbances, depigmentation and hair loss. It is very toxic in overdose
b) False – Recognized with pyrimethamine with sulfadoxine
c) True – Also potentiates the bradycardic effect of beta blockers
d) False
e) True – In glucose 6-phosphate dehydrogenase-deficient patients

347 a) True
b) True
c) False – A single dose of praziquantel is curative
d) True – Pyrantel is also effective
e) False – Diethylcarbamazine, in addition corticosteroids may be needed to treat allergic reactions to dying larvae

348 a) True Nausea and vomiting are often the principal immediate
b) False toxic effects associated with cytotoxic chemotherapy. To
c) False avoid tissue necrosis, another immediate effect, expert
d) False attention to vascular access is mandatory
e) True

349 a) True There are two patterns of bone marrow recovery after
b) True suppression: rapid and delayed. The use of haematopoietic
c) True growth factors, e.g. erythropoietin, G-CSF is a major
d) False advance in supportive care. Vincristine and bleomycin
e) False seldom cause myelosuppression. Vincristine is associated with peripheral or autonomic neuropathy. It is very irritant and must never be given into the intrathecal space. Extravasation from a vein causes profound local ulceration

350 a) True Broad-spectrum antibacterial treatment must be started
b) True empirically in febrile neutropenic patients without waiting
c) False for culture results. The effect on fertility and the risk of
d) True future fetal abnormalities are very variable. Alkylating
e) True agents are particularly harmful. Successful pregnancies are not unusual in women at least six months after completion of chemotherapy. Sperm and oocyte storage should be considered

351 a) True Cyclophosphamide is used as part of combination
b) True chemotherapy for various lymphomas and leukaemias
c) True and in myeloma. It is similarly used in treating certain

d) True   solid tumours (e.g. breast cancer, small cell lung cancer).
e) True   In cytotoxic doses it is usually given by intravenous injection

352 a) True
b) True
c) False   – Contraindicated in significant renal impairment, excreted primarily in the urine
d) True
e) True

353 a) False   – Peripheral neuropathy is common with vincristine
b) True   – Etoposide, a topoisomerase II inhibitor, is particularly active in small cell lung cancer
c) True
d) True   – Irinotecan is a topoisomerase I inhibitor
e) False   – Pulmonary fibrosis is associated with busulfan or bleomycin therapy

354 a) True   Cisplatin is of value in metastatic germ cell cancers
b) True   (seminoma and teratoma). Carboplatin is widely used
c) False   in advanced ovarian cancer and lung cancer (especially
d) True   in small cell lung cancer). It is generally better tolerated
e) True   than cisplatin; however it is more myelosuppressive. Oxaliplatin is used in metastatic colorectal cancer in combination with fluorouracil and folinic acid. Neurotoxicity is dose limiting

355 a) True   Paclitaxel was derived from the bark of the Pacific yew
b) False   tree. It antagonizes the depolymerization of microtubules,
c) True   halting mitosis. The affected cells undergo apoptosis.
d) True   Hypersensitivity reactions, bone marrow suppression,
e) False   myalgia, arthralgia, nausea and vomiting and alopecia are also associated adverse effects

356 a) False   – Use parenteral iron. Erythropoietin treatment will precipitate iron deficiency and generally supplemental iron should be prescribed concomitantly with erythropoietin
b) False
c) True
d) True
e) False

357 a) True   – Often self-administered
b) True
c) False   – Increases proliferation of the malignant clone
d) True
e) True   – Also myalgia, fever, splenomegaly, thrombocytopenia and abnormal hepatic transaminases

358 a) True – Fat redistribution, insulin resistance and dyslipidaemia
b) True
c) True
d) False – Associated with nucleoside reverse transcriptase inhibitors
e) True – Via inhibition of CYP3A, increasing the risk of rifabutin toxicity

EMQ ANSWERS

359 ANTIBACTERIAL DRUGS

1 E Lyme disease: doxycycline.

2 G Invasive salmonellosis: ciprofloxacin or cefotaxime.

3 A Antibiotic-associated colitis (pseudomembranous colitis): oral metronidazole or oral vancomycin.

4 H Peritonitis in a patient allergic to cephalosporins: gentamicin + metronidazole.

5 D Uncomplicated community-acquired pneumonia in a penicillin-allergic patient: clarithromycin

360 ANTIBACTERIAL DRUGS

1 A Severe community-acquired pneumonia: cefuroxime and clarithromycin (add flucloxacillin if staphylococcal infection suspected).

2 H Acute septic arthritis: flucloxacillin and sodium fusidate.

3 D Suspected bacterial meningitis in a 25-year-old woman: ceftriaxone.

4 C Bacterial endocarditis following dental extraction: benzylpenicillin and gentamicin.

5 F Pyelonephritis (beta-lactam allergic): ciprofloxacin.

361 HIV

1 D Zidovudine (ZDV, AZT) undergoes intracellular anabolic phosphorylation to its triphosphate anabolite (ZDV-TP) which acts as a competitive inhibitor to endogenous nucleotides for the HIV-reverse transcriptase. ZDV-TP similarly competitively inhibits the mitochondrial DNA polymerase gamma. ZDV is used as one of the component drugs in highly active anti-retroviral therapy (HAART). Other compounds in this group called the nucleoside reverse transcriptase inhibitors

(NRTIs) include lamivudine (3TC), stavudine (d4T), ddI, emtricitabine and abacavir. The commonest toxicities of ZDV are fatigue, anaemia and gastrointestinal upset.

2 **F** Enfuvirtide is a peptide which blocks the interaction between the HIV gp41 protein and the host cell membrane by binding to a hydrophobic groove in the N36 region of gp41. Due to its unique mechanism of action, enfurvitide is active against HIV which has developed resistance to HAART. It is given by intravenous injection and its main side-effects are infusion reactions, lymphadenopathy, flu-like syndrome and eosinophilia.

3 **C** Efavirenz is a non-nucleoside (non-competitive) HIV reverse transcriptase (HIV-RT) inhibitor (NNRTI) which binds to an allosteric (non-catalytic) site on HIV-RT, inhibiting its function. Other drugs in this class are nevirapine and delaverdine. They are synergistic with NRTIs against HIV-RT. They should not be used as monotherapy as viral resistance develops quickly and are thus a component of HAART. The main side-effects are gastrointestinal upsets, lipodystrophy, arthralgia, myalgia and complex drug–drug interactions due to modulation of CYP450.

4 **A** Azatanavir is a competitive inhibitor of the HIV protease and inhibits the cleavage of HIV pre-proteins into active HIV proteins. It is one of a class of HIV protease inhibitors that is most potent in inhibiting HIV replication. Other agents in the class include amprenavir (fosamprenavir), ritonavir, indinavir, lopinavir, nelfinavir, saquinavir and tripanavir. These agents form part of HAART. Side-effects include gastrointestinal upset, fatigue, lipodystrophy, hyperglycaemia–hypertriglyceridaemia and drug–drug interactions by inhibiting CYP3A.

5 **G** Raltegravir. This is a competitive inhibitor of the insertion of HIV DNA into the host genome of the enzyme HIV integrase. It is also termed a strandtransfer inhibitor. It is administered orally on a twice-daily basis and is only to be used in patients who have resistance to standard HAART combinations. Common toxicities are diarrhoea, nausea, headaches and myositis.

362 HIV

1 **J** Foscarnet is a pyrophosphate analogue which is a non-competitive inhibitor of CMV DNA polymerase and HIV-RT. It thus can inhibit replication of both viruses. It is primarily used to treat CMV infections. It is administered systemically and its main side-effects are nephrotoxicity, CNS irritability, hypocalcaemia and hypomagnesaemia.

2 **D** Zidovudine (ZDV, AZT) undergoes intracellular anabolic phosphorylation to its triphosphate anabolite (ZDV-TP) which acts as a competitive inhibitor to endogenous nucleotides for the HIV-RT. ZDV-TP similarly competitively inhibits the mitochondrial DNA polymerase gamma.

The anaemia it causes is macrocytic (with normal B_{12} and folate) and impaired erythroid precursor development manifested as reticulocytopenia. Aplastic anaemia can be observed, as can suppression of the myeloid lineages (neutropenia). This effect is dose-dependent and minimized by treatment with erythropoietin.

3 G Ritonavir is one of the least potent HIV-protease inhibitors used to treat HIV. One of its ancilliary properties is that it is a potent inhibitor of CYP3A (gastrointestinal and hepatic) and the drug efflux protein in the gastrointestinal tract P-glycoprotein (MDR-1/ABC-B1). By inhibiting the function of both these proteins low-dose ritonavir is used in combination with other agents in this drug class (e.g. lopinavir) to enhance their bioavailability. This is termed 'boosted' lopinavir therapy.

4 H Tenofovir is the first nucleotide (as distinct from nucleoside – a non-phosphorylated purine or pyrimidine) reverse transcriptase inhibitor and is used in combination with NRTIs. It is a derivative of adenosine monophosphate, but lacks the ribose ring. It undergoes further sequential phosphorylation to the diphosphate and then the triphosphate which is a competitive inhibitor of HIV-RT.

5 A Lopinavir – see explanation for answer 3 G above.

363 MALARIA AND PARASITIC INFECTIONS

1 B Quinine sulphate is the drug of choice for treating an acute attack of falciparum malaria where the parasite is likely to be chloroquine resistant.

2 A Atovaquone and proguanil is a recommended prophylactic antimalarial for a visit to Ghana (high risk of malaria, widespread chloroquine resistance).

3 C Primaquine is used after standard choloroquine therapy to eradicate hepatic forms of *P. vivax* and *P. malariae*.

4 F Mebendazole is appropriate for treating threadworm infection in those over 2 years. It is also effective in roundworm, whipworm and hookworm infections. Piperazine may be used in threadworm and roundworm infections from the age of three months.

5 J Metronidazole is the treatment of choice for giardiasis and acute invasive amoebic dysentery.

364 CANCER

1 A Imatinib is the first in class oral targeted therapy for Philadelphia chromosome-positive chronic myeloid leukaemia (CML). It is an ATP mimetic and binds to the ATP site of the BCR-Abl fusion protein and acts as a competitive inhibitor of this kinase enzyme in the leukaemic cells.

2 C Irinotecan is a compound of the camtothecin family. It is an inhibitor of the DNA topisomerase I which locks the DNA in the cleavable complex, preventing replication. Its metabolite SN-38 is the most active moiety at inhibiting DNA topoisomerase.

3 E Trastuzumab is a humanized monoclonal antibody that binds to the extracellular non-ligand-binding domain of HER2/NEU (EGFR-2) with a K_d in the nanomolar range. This target is overexpressed on a number of neoplastic cells, especially breast cancers and prevents signal transduction and proliferation.

4 J Bevacizumab is a humanized monoclonal antibody that binds to VEGF A, B and C, preventing their subsequent interaction with the VEGF receptor on new vessel walls in the tumour neovasculature and thus preventing tumour angiogenesis. It has activity in colon, lung and renal cell carcinoma.

5 H Gefitinib is the first in class oral EGFR-targeted therapy. It is an ATP mimetic and inhibits the tyrosine kinase found on the EGF receptor, which autophosphorylates the receptor and thus yields signal transduction and cellular proliferation. Inhibition of this signalling leads to apoptosis and cell death. Many epithelial tumours overexpress this receptor – lung, head and neck and breast cancer.

365 CANCER

1 E Interferon is used in cancer therapy in high doses to treat metastatic renal carcinoma and melanoma. Common side-effects include fatigue, a flu-like syndrome, memory impairment, hyperglycaemia, bone marrow suppression and hypothyroidism.

2 C Fludarabine is used in combination therapy for acute leukaemias. It commonly causes neurotoxicity which includes a reversible cerebellar syndrome. This is similar to the toxicity caused by cytarabine (cytosine arabinoside). Other common toxicities include haematopoietic suppression.

3 B Clinically available platinum compounds (cisplatin, carboplatin and oxaliplatin) are active as part of combination chemotherapy in many solid tumours. Cisplatin and carboplatin commonly produce renal tubular dysfunction which may lead to tubular necrosis, which is cumulative and may in some cases be only partially reversible. Oxaliplatin causes least nephrotoxicity. Hydration, electrolyte replacement and diuresis minimize the platinum compound tubular toxicity, which is a direct concentration-dependent toxic effect on tubular cells.

4 D Interleukin 2 is used to treat metastatic melanoma and renal carcinoma. It stimulates the immune response against tumour cells. Interleukin 2 itself and the other cytokines that it releases produce a pulmonary capillary leak syndrome and acute respiratory distress syndrome (ARDS), which is reversible but may require ventilatory support.

5 H Sorafenib is effective in treating advanced renal cell carcinoma and inhibits Raf kinase and the VEGFR tyrosine kinase. Almost all the agents which target VEGF or the VEGF tyrosine kinase inhibitor can produce hypertension in patients who were previously normotensive or exacerbate hypertension in patients with high blood pressure. The mechanism of this effect is unclear. Treatment with calcium channel blockers and/or ACE inhibitors can ameliorate this side-effect.

CHAPTER NINE

CLINICAL IMMUNOPHARMACOLOGY

MULTIPLE CHOICE QUESTIONS

366 Glucocorticosteroids inhibit:

a) Platelet thromboxane A_2 synthesis
b) Histamine release
c) Leukotriene C_4 and D_4 synthesis
d) Arachidonic acid metabolism
e) Transcription of tumour necrosis factor (TNF) and interleukin 6 (IL-6)

367 The following agents are used to prevent or treat graft-versus-host disease:

a) Methylprednisolone
b) Ciclosporin
c) Mycophenolate mofetil
d) Tacrolimus
e) Infliximab

368 Adverse effects associated with ciclosporin include:

a) Reduced glomerular filtration pressure leading to nephrotoxicity
b) Gingival hyperplasia
c) Alopecia
d) Tremor
e) Hypokalaemia

369 Administration of basiliximab (IL-2 receptor blocking antibody) may cause the following side-effects:

a) Hypotension
b) Delayed, severe dyspnoea and wheezing
c) Fever and chills
d) Aseptic meningitis
e) Cardiomyopathy

370 Mycophenolate mofetil:

a) Is a prodrug
b) Inhibits inosine monophosphate dehydrogenase, impairing *de novo* purine synthesis in T and B cells
c) Is given intravenously
d) Causes leukopenia
e) Is used as adjunct therapy in solid organ transplantation and is more effective than azathioprine

371 Natalizumab is indicated in the treatment of refractory:

a) Rheumatoid arthritis
b) Eczema
c) Asthma
d) Multiple sclerosis
e) Acute solid organ transplant rejection

372 The following agents inhibit the metabolism of ciclosporin:

a) Diltiazem
b) Itraconazole
c) Cimetidine
d) Rifampicin
e) Gentamicin

373 The following are indicated in the management of acute anaphylactic shock following a bee sting out of hospital and without monitoring facilities:

a) Intramuscular adrenaline (epinephrine) (0.5–1 mL, 1 in 1000)
b) Intravenous adrenaline (epinephrine) (10 mL, 1 in 10 000)
c) Intravenous hydrocortisone
d) Intravenous chlorpheniramine
e) Oxygen

374 Azathioprine:

a) Is metabolized to 6-mercaptopurine
b) Inhibits delayed hypersensitivity (cell-mediated immunity) and those aspects of inflammation that require cell division
c) Is administered by continuous infusion
d) Causes neutropenia and thrombocytopenia
e) Concurrent allopurinol increases the clearance of azathioprine

375 Cyclophosphamide is used as an immunosuppressive in the following diseases:
   a) Pneumoconiosis (silicosis)
   b) Autoimmune haemolytic anaemia
   c) Nephrotic syndrome with minimal microscopic glomerular changes
   d) Nephritis due to systemic lupus erythematosus
   e) Wegener's granulomatosis

376 Fexofenadine:
   a) Is a competitive antagonist at the H_1 receptor
   b) Is used as a sedative in children
   c) Is effective treatment for motion sickness
   d) Is used prophylactically in hayfever
   e) Plasma concentrations when very high can lead to prolonged QTc and torsades de pointes

377 The following are successfully used in the management of allergic rhinitis (hayfever):
   a) Oral H_3 receptor antagonists
   b) Desensitization with a mix of grass pollen, cat dander and house dust mite
   c) Nasal sodium cromoglicate
   d) Nasal terbutaline
   e) Nasal budesonide

378 Annual immunization with influenza vaccine is strongly recommended for individuals aged over six months with the following conditions:
   a) Immunosuppression because of prolonged corticosteroid treatment
   b) Diabetes mellitus requiring insulin or oral hypoglycaemic drugs
   c) Patients with chronic lung disease
   d) Human immunodeficiency virus (HIV) infection
   e) Chronic renal disease

Answers: see pages 163–165

EXTENDED MATCHING QUESTIONS

379 CLINICAL IMMUNOPHARMACOLOGY

A	Tacrolimus	F	Natalizumab
B	Mycophenolate	G	Etanercept
C	Muromonab	H	Basilixumab
D	Prednisolone	I	Azathioprine
E	Aldesleukin (IL-2)	J	Methotrexate

Match a drug from the list above which corresponds most closely to the statement below:

1 An anti-IL-2 receptor antibody
2 Toxicity can be reduced by 'folinic acid rescue'
3 A calcineurin inhibitor that is more potent than ciclosporin
4 An anti-$\alpha_4\beta_3$ integrin monoclonal antibody used in patients with progressive multiple sclerosis
5 Used in metastatic renal cell carcinoma

380 CLINICAL IMMUNOPHARMACOLOGY

A	Nedocromil	F	Sirolimus
B	6-Mercaptopurine	G	Ciclosporin
C	Natalizumab	H	Methylprednisolone
D	Fexofenadine	I	Mycophenolate mofetil
E	Meningococcal vaccine	J	Basilixumab

Match the single agent most correctly linked with each of the following pharmacodynamic effects:

1 Gingival hyperplasia
2 Inhbition of mammalian target of rapamycin (mTOR)
3 Hypokalaemia
4 Thrombocytopenia
5 Binds to the $\alpha_4\beta_3$ integrin

ANSWERS: see pages 165–166

MCQ ANSWERS **163**

ANSWERS

MCQ ANSWERS

366
a) False   Glucocorticosteroids reduce the transcription of
b) True   proinflammatory mediators (e.g. TNF, IL-6) and inhibit
c) True   type I, II, III and IV hypersensitivity reactions. They are the
d) True   most widely used immunosuppressive agents. They inhibit
e) True   eicosanoid synthesis from arachidonic acid in nucleated
            cells by increasing the production of lipocortin, an inhibitor
            of phospholipase A_2 (PLA$_2$)

367
a) True
b) True   – Specific T lymphocyte suppressor, primarily against T
            helper cells
c) True   – Need regular blood counts
d) True   – Is neurotoxic and nephrotoxic
e) True   – Monoclonal antibody which binds TNF and prevents its
            action

368
a) True   – Also may cause hypertension. Nephrotoxicity may be
            reduced by concurrent calcium channel blockade
b) True
c) False   – Hirsutism
d) True   – May be an early sign of toxic plasma concentrations
e) False   – Causes hyperkalaemia

369
a) True   – Any murine/humanized monoclonal antibody when given
            to humans may cause anaphylaxis
b) True   – Manifestation of a delayed hypersensitivity reaction
c) True
d) False   – Intravenous human normal immunoglobulin (HNIG) in
            high dose can cause this
e) False

370
a) True   – It is a prodrug ester of mycophenolic acid; the latter under-
            goes hepatic glucuronidation to an inactive metabolite
b) True   – Blocks purine synthesis in proliferating lymphocytes and
            may reduce production of proinflammatory cytokines
c) False   – Is given orally. Antacids decrease its absorption. Also
            causes gastrointestinal side-effects
d) True
e) True

371
a) False   Natalizumab is an anti-$\alpha_4\beta_3$ integrin monoclonal antibody.
b) False   It inhibits the migration/trafficking of leukocytes into the

     c) False   CNS. Its use in severe progressive multiple sclerosis was
     d) True   temporarily suspended due to an association with
     e) False   progressive multifocal leukoencephalopathy (PML)

372 a) True   CYP3A4 inhibitors block ciclosporin (and tacrolimus)
     b) True   metabolism, increasing the risk of toxicity if the dose of
     c) True   immunosuppressant is not reduced
     d) False   – Rifampicin (and all rifamycins) induce CYP3A4, reducing
                    ciclosporin blood concentrations for the same dose
     e) False   – But gentamicin potentiates the nephrotoxicity of
                    ciclosporin

373 a) True   – Life saving
     b) False   – May induce ventricular fibrillation
     c) True   – But takes 4–6 hours to be of benefit
     d) False   – The use of intravenous antihistamines here is controversial
     e) True   – If hypotensive, intravenous fluids may also be of value and
                    may be available in an ambulance

374 a) True   Azathioprine is an antimetabolite and thus most effective
     b) True   on proliferating cells. It is administered by mouth and
     c) False   metabolized to its active moiety – 6-mercaptopurine. It is
     d) True   used as an adjunct to prevent transplant rejection and also
     e) False   in the treatment of autoimmune diseases such as systemic
                    lupus erythematosus and chronic active hepatitis. Owing to
                    its potential toxicity (bone marrow) it is usually reserved
                    for situations in which corticosteroids alone are inadequate

375 a) False   Cyclophosphamide, in addition to its use as a cytotoxic
     b) False   cancer drug, is particularly valuable in aggressive
     c) True   autoimmune diseases inhibiting lymphocyte proliferation
     d) True
     e) True

376 a) True
     b) False   – Fexofenadine, cetirizine and loratadine are 'non-sedative'
                    antihistamines
     c) False
     d) True
     e) False   – Fexofenadine is the non-cardiotoxic metabolite of terfenadine

377 a) False   Avoidance of allergens is ideal but rarely practical. With the
     b) False   exception of oral H_1 blockers, local therapy is preferred. If
     c) True   indicated, desensitization therapy with a single allergen is
     d) False   acceptable, but the risk of anaphylaxis is high and it should
     e) True   only be undertaken in specialist allergy clinics

378 a) True   Influenza viruses are constantly changing their antigenic
     b) True   structure. Current influenza vaccines are grown in chick
     c) True   embryos and are contraindicated in those with
     d) True   hypersensitivity to eggs
     e) True

EMQ ANSWERS

379 CLINICAL IMMUNOPHARMACOLOGY

1 H Basilixumab is an anti-IL-2 receptor antibody which inhibits IL-2-mediated T-cell activation and is used in the management of organ transplant rejection.

2 J Methotrexate resembles folic acid and competes with it at the active site of dihydrofolate reductase. Consequently methotrexate blocks nucleic acid synthesis. It is used as an immunosuppressant and anticancer drug. Folinic acid circumvents the block and can minimize bone marrow and gut toxicity, whilst maintaining efficacy if administered at a set time after methotrexate administration.

3 A Tacrolimus is often used in patients who are refractory to ciclosporin. Wide interindividual variation exists in its pharmacokinetics. It is metabolized by CYP3A4. It may cause more neurotoxicity and nephrotoxicity than ciclosporin. Therapeutic monitoring of trough drug concentrations is useful.

4 F Natalizumab inhibits leukocyte migration into the CNS and is licensed for use in highly active multiple sclerosis. There is an association with opportunistic infection including (rarely) PML.

5 E Aldesleukin (recombinant IL-2) is licensed for metastatic renal cell carcinoma.

380 CLINICAL IMMUNOPHARMACOLOGY

1 G Ciclosporin causes gingival hyperplasia in 4–16 per cent of recipients. It is reversible and appears more common in paediatric patients. Few drugs cause this side-effect and others include phenytoin and nifedipine.

2 F Sirolimus (also known as rapamycin) binds to the mammalias target of Rapamycin (mTOR) and inhibits mTOR-mediated mitogenic signal transduction.

3 H Methylprednisolone and most synthetic glucocorticosteroids cause hypokalaemia as they have some mineralocorticoid action and thus promote potassium loss via the kidney.

4 B 6-Mercaptopurine causes bone marrow suppression, especially thrombocytopenia, but also neutropenia.

5 C Natalizumab binds to the endothelial cell adhesion molecule $\alpha_4\beta_3$ integrin. Thus it impairs migration of inflammatory cells, especially lymphocytes, from the vascular space into the tissues. It is used in progressive multiple sclerosis.

CHAPTER TEN

THE SKIN AND THE EYE

MULTIPLE CHOICE QUESTIONS

381 Acne vulgaris:
- **a)** Can be effectively treated with topical benzoyl peroxide
- **b)** May be precipitated by oral methylprednisolone
- **c)** Is caused by propionibacteria
- **d)** Cold tar treatment reduces the severity of lesions
- **e)** Can be exacerbated by oral aciclovir

382 Isotretinoin:
- **a)** Is a synthetic vitamin D analogue
- **b)** The usual course of treatment is two weeks
- **c)** Is teratogenic
- **d)** Causes hirsutism
- **e)** Is eliminated from the body over a period of weeks

383 The following are effective in the management of eczema:
- **a)** Topical betamethasone
- **b)** Topical alpha-tocopherol
- **c)** Dithranol
- **d)** Calcipotriol
- **e)** Emulsifying ointment

384 Local application of the following are of benefit in the management of psoriasis:
- **a)** Adepalene
- **b)** Salicylic acid
- **c)** Psoralens
- **d)** Dithranol
- **e)** Calcipotriol

385 The following may be effective in the management of severe psoriasis:
a) Weekly methotrexate
b) Erythromycin
c) Efalizumab
d) Nateglinide
e) Acitretin

386 The following drugs are recognized causes of Stevens–Johnson syndrome:
a) Co-trimoxazole
b) Amoxicillin
c) L-Thyroxine
d) Phenytoin
e) Lamotrigine

387 The following infections/infestations are paired with their appropriate treatment:
a) Candida vulvovaginitis – topical ketoconazole
b) Fungal nail infections – oral griseofulvin
c) Tinea corporis – topical clotrimazole
d) Initial or recurrent genital herpes simplex – oral aciclovir
e) Scabies – topical malathion

388 Administration of the following eye drops/ointments can produce the correctly paired systemic effects:
a) Carteolol – bradycardia
b) Aciclovir – alopecia
c) Gentamicin – renal tubular necrosis
d) Prednisolone – hypercalcaemia
e) Pilocarpine – dry mouth

389 Dilatation of the pupil (mydriasis) is produced by:
a) Cyclopentolate
b) Dorzolamide
c) Atropine
d) Phenylephrine
e) Ketorolac

390 In the treatment of open angle glaucoma the following drugs are effective:
a) Acetozolamide
b) Chlorpheniramine
c) Dexamethasone
d) Latanoprost
e) Timolol

391 The following treatments have been correctly paired with their licensed indication in ophthalmology:

a) Aciclovir – cytomegalovirus (CMV) retinitis

b) Ranizumab – age-related macular degeneration

c) Ciprofloxacin – corneal ulceration

d) Fusidic acid – hypersensitivity reactions

e) Travoprost – open angle glaucoma

Answers: see pages 171–172

EXTENDED MATCHING QUESTIONS

392 DRUGS AND THE SKIN

A	Calcipotriol	F	Methotrexate
B	Lindane 1 per cent	G	Prednisolone
C	Terbinafine	H	Retinoic acid
D	Clotrimizole	I	Topical minoxidil
E	Topical aciclovir	J	Low-dose doxycycline

Match the most appropriate drug from the list above with the indication below:

1 Topical treatment for acne
2 Topical treatment for psoriasis
3 Systemic treatment for refractory psoriasis
4 Tinea pedis
5 Fungal nail infection

393 DRUGS AND THE EYE

A	Tropicamide	F	Ganciclovir
B	Mannitol	G	Pilocarpine
C	Fusidic acid	H	Timolol
D	Betamethasone	I	Rifampicin
E	Aciclovir	J	Verteporfin

Match the indication/effect from the list below with the most appropriate drug:

1 Causes miosis
2 CMV retinitis
3 Acute glaucoma
4 Short-duration mydriatic
5 Discolours soft contact lenses

ANSWERS: see page 173

ANSWERS

MCQ ANSWERS

381
a) True   Acne vulgaris occurs in at least 90 per cent of adolescents.
b) True   The topical use of peeling agents such as benzoyl peroxide
c) True   or azelaic acid or topical retinoids on a regular basis is
d) False   usually all that is necessary. In more severe cases oral
e) False   antibacterial drugs are beneficial and if this is ineffective
                 oral isotretinoin may be considered by specialists

382
a) False   Isotretinoin is a vitamin A analogue. It is prescribed under
b) False   hospital supervision usually for at least four months. There is
c) True   a persistent risk of teratogenicity for at least one month after
d) False   stopping oral therapy. Co-pyrindiol (cyproterone acetate, an
e) True   anti-androgen with ethinylestradiol) is useful in women
                 whose acne is refractory to antibiotics/topical treatments and
                 who also wish to receive oral contraception. There is an
                 increased risk of thromboembolism

383
a) True   In mild wet eczema, the topical use of drying agents such
b) False   as lotions of aluminium acetate or calamine are useful.
c) False   When the lesions are dry and scaly the use of emollients
d) False   (e.g. E45) combined with a keratolytic is beneficial.
e) True   Topical corticosteroids are often required both in 'wet' and
                 'dry' eczema. Nocturnal pruritus may be relieved by
                 sedative antihistamines

384
a) False   – Adapalene is a topical retinoid-like drug used in mild to
                 moderate acne
b) True   – Enhances rate of loss of surface scale
c) False   – PUVA (photochemotherapy using an oral psoralen with
                 long-wave ultraviolet radiation) is an effective treatment
                 for psoriasis
d) True   – Irritates normal skin
e) True   – Does not irritate normal skin

385
a) True   – Folic acid reduces the possibility of toxicity
b) False   – Sometimes useful in acne
c) True   – Inhibits T-cell activation
d) False   – Used in type 2 diabetes in combination with metformin
e) True   – An oral retinoid

386
a) True   All sulfonamides and beta-lactam antibacterials can cause
b) True   this syndrome
c) False

    d) True
    e) True

387 a) True   – With unusual/recurrent skin infections consider diabetes mellitus or immunosuppression. Antibiotic therapy, diabetes mellitus and immunosuppression are risk factors
    b) True
    c) True
    d) True
    e) True

388 a) True   – Intraocular administered doses avoid hepatic first-pass metabolism and can lead to bradycardia
    b) False
    c) False   – Not enough absorbed to cause systemic toxicity
    d) False
    e) True   – With high doses enough can be absorbed to produce systemic anticholinergic effects

389 a) True   – Muscarinic (M_3 in the eye) receptor antagonist blocks action of sphincter muscle of the iris
    b) False   – Topical carbonic anhydrase inhibitor
    c) True   – Muscarinic (M_3 in the eye) receptor antagonist blocks action of sphincter muscle of the iris
    d) True   – Stimulates α_1 adrenoreceptors constricting the radial muscle of the iris
    e) False   – Non-steroidal anti-inflammatory drug (NSAID) used in eye drops for prophylaxis and reduction of inflammation following ocular surgery

390 a) True   – Carbonic anhydrase inhibitor given systemically reduces production of the aqueous humour
    b) False   – First-generation antihistamine which will dilate the pupil (due to its anticholinergic properties), worsening glaucoma
    c) False   – Steroids can exacerbate glaucoma in certain genetically predisposed patients
    d) True   – Prostaglandin $F_{2\alpha}$ analogue lowers intraocular pressure by increasing uveoscleral flow
    e) True   – Beta-adrenergic antagonist reduces secretion/formation of aqueous humour

391 a) False   – Aciclovir is indicated for herpes simplex infection
    b) True   – Blocks vascular endothelial growth factor (VEGF)
    c) True
    d) False   – Useful for staphylococcal infections
    e) True   – Prostaglandin analogue which increases uveoscleral flow

392 DRUGS AND THE SKIN

1 H The topical use of keratolytic agents such as benzoyl peroxide or retinoic acid on a regular basis in conjunction with systemic antibiotic therapy is successful in most patients with acne.

2 A Calcipotriol, a vitamin D analogue, is effective topically in psoriasis.

3 F Immunosuppressants such as ciclosporin or methotrexate are sometimes required in refractory psoriasis.

4 D Topical clotrimazole is effective in fungal skin infections.

5 C Terbinafine is the treatment of choice for fungal nail infections.

393 DRUGS AND THE EYE

1 G Pilocarpine, a cholinergic agonist, constricts the pupil and is used in simple glaucoma topically.

2 F Ganciclovir (foscarnet is an alternative) can be used via the intravenous/intraocular route to treat CMV retinitis.

3 B Acute glaucoma is a medical emergency. Intravenous mannitol, an osmotic diuretic, shifts water from intracellular and transcellular compartments (including the eye) into plasma and promotes fluid loss via diuresis. In addition a carbonic anhydrase inhibitor (intravenous acetazolamide or topical dorzolamide) may be required.

4 A Tropicamide is a convenient short-acting topical mydriatic frequently used to assist examination of the fundus.

5 I Rifampicin discolours urine, saliva, tears and other body secretions orange-red.

CHAPTER ELEVEN

CLINICAL TOXICOLOGY

MULTIPLE CHOICE QUESTIONS

394 Methadone:
  a) Has the potential to cause dependence
  b) Can only be prescribed to registered addicts by doctors with a special licence
  c) Is usually administered as an elixir
  d) Depresses the cough centre
  e) Effects are reversed by naloxone

395 The following are clinical signs consistent with heroin (diamorphine) intoxication:
  a) Hypertension
  b) Rapid respiratory rate
  c) Hypothermia
  d) Pinpoint pupils
  e) Slurred speech

396 Features of the opioid withdrawal syndrome include:
  a) Yawning
  b) Rhinorrhoea
  c) Mydriasis
  d) Diarrhoea
  e) Tremor

397 Specific causes of death which are positively related to smoking include:
  a) Ischaemic heart disease
  b) Cancer of the oesophagus
  c) Emphysema
  d) Aortic aneurysm
  e) Cancer of the tongue

398 There is an increased rate of metabolism of the following drugs in smokers:
   a) Diazepam
   b) Phenytoin
   c) Ethanol
   d) Warfarin
   e) Theophylline

399 Ethyl alcohol (ethanol):
   a) The majority of oral ethanol is absorbed from the small intestine
   b) Ethanol delays gastic emptying
   c) 95 per cent of ingested ethanol is metabolized
   d) Ethanol elimination demonstrates first-order kinetics
   e) Is second to heroin as the most important drug of dependence in Western Europe

400 Cardiovascular complications associated with alcohol consumption include:
   a) Atrial fibrillation
   b) Buerger's disease
   c) Cardiomyopathy
   d) Coronary artery disease
   e) Peripheral vascular disease

401 Delirium tremens:
   a) Occurs in approximately 60 per cent of patients withdrawing from alcohol
   b) Has a mortality of 5–10 per cent
   c) Benzodiazepines are contraindicated
   d) Thiamine should be administered parenterally
   e) Phenytoin should be administered prophylactically to prevent convulsions

402 Chronic use of anabolic steroids is associated with:
   a) Pancreatitis
   b) Ototoxicity
   c) Hepatic tumours
   d) Cardiomyopathy
   e) Peripheral neuropathy

403 3,4-Methylenedioxy-*N*-methylamphetamine (MDMA or ecstasy):
a) Has agonist properties at the 5HT$_2$ receptor
b) Has mixed hallucinogenic and stimulant properties
c) Occasionally causes hyperpyrexia
d) In chronic use has been associated with increased impulsivity and impaired memory
e) Chronic usage may cause irreversible degeneration of serotonergic nerves

404 The combination of coma, dilated pupils, hyperreflexia and tachycardia is consistent with overdose of the following drugs when taken alone:
a) Co-dydramol
b) Dosulepin
c) Aspirin
d) Amitriptyline
e) Lorazepam

405 The following suspected overdoses are indications for emergency measurement of drug concentration:
a) Iron
b) Methanol
c) Amitriptyline
d) Temazepam
e) Salicylates

406 The following poisons/drugs have been correctly paired with an appropriate antidote/specific measure:
a) Paracetamol – acetylcysteine
b) Iron – desferrioxamine
c) Codeine – naloxone
d) Organophosphorus insecticides – dicobalt edetate
e) Methanol – ethanol

407 An 18-year-old woman is admitted 4 hours after taking 50 paracetamol and 50 × 300 mg aspirin tablets. The following statements are correct:
a) She is likely to be in a grade IV coma
b) Stomach washout is indicated
c) Acetylcysteine should be administered
d) Blood gases are likely to show a mixed metabolic acidosis/respiratory alkalosis
e) If petechiae and subconjunctival haemorrhages are present, fresh frozen plasma should be administered immediately

408 The following are confirmed aphrodisiacs:
- **a)** Ginseng
- **b)** Oysters
- **c)** Extract of rhino horn
- **d)** Passion fruit
- **e)** Vitamin E

Answers: see pages 179–182

EXTENDED MATCHING QUESTIONS

409 CLINICAL MANIFESTATIONS OF DRUG OVERDOSE

A	Amitriptyline		F	Iron
B	Simvastatin		G	Aspirin
C	Lithium		H	Methadone
D	MDMA (ecstasy)		I	Atenolol
E	Temazepam		J	Nifedipine

Choose the drug overdose from the list above which is most likely to present with the symptoms/signs listed below:

1   Coma, hypotension, flaccidity
2   Coma, pinpoint pupils, hypoventilation
3   Coma, dilated pupils, hyperreflexia, tachycardia
4   Restlessness, hypertonia, hyperreflexia, pyrexia
5   Tinnitus, overbreathing, pyrexia, sweating, flushing, usually alert

410 ANTIDOTES/OTHER SPECIFIC MEASURES IN THE MANAGEMENT OF POISONING

A	Acetylcysteine		G	Calcium chloride
B	Desferrioxamine		H	Flumazenil
C	Ethanol		I	Urinary alkalisation
D	Dimercaprol (BAL)		J	Oxygen, intravenous sodium nitrite followed by intravenous sodium thiosulphate
E	Naloxone			
F	Pralidoxime			

Match the most appropriate antidote/other specific measure from the above list to treat a clinically significant overdose with the agent listed below:

1   Aspirin
2   Paracetamol
3   Methanol
4   Iron
5   Cyanide

ANSWERS: see pages 182–183

ANSWERS

MCQ ANSWERS

394 a) True
  b) False
  c) True
  d) True
  e) True

Methadone elixir/mixture is the mainstay of many drug addiction clinics. It has a long half-life of 15–55 hours and it is very difficult to administer these oral formulations as an injection. Doctors should report cases of drug misuse to their regional or national drug misuse data base or centre (see BNF)

395 a) False
  b) False
  c) True
  d) True
  e) True

Initially intravenous heroin produces an intense euphoria for several seconds (often accompanied by nausea/ vomiting). Many chronic users often claim the only effect is remission from abstinence symptoms

396 a) True
  b) True
  c) True
  d) True
  e) True

Withdrawal symptoms generally start at the time the next dose would usually be given and their intensity is related to the usual dose. For heroin, symptoms usually reach a maximum at 36–72 hours and gradually subside over the next 5–10 days. Lofexidine, an α_2 antagonist, alleviates many of the withdrawal symptoms. Loperamide helps reduce the diarrhoea

397 a) True
  b) True
  c) True
  d) True
  e) True

In the UK, in men under 70 years, the ratio of death rate among cigarette smokers to non-smokers is 2:1. To assist smokers to give up, nicotine chewing gum, patches, sublingual tablets and spray are available. Varenicline, a selective nicotine receptor partial agonist, and bupropion, an antidepressant, have been introduced as adjuncts to smoking cessation. Bupropion is contraindicated in patients with a history of seizures or of eating disorders

398 a) False
  b) False
  c) False
  d) False
  e) True

In addition to pharmacokinetic differences, smokers may exhibit altered pharmacodynamic responses (e.g. smokers show less CNS depression after a standard dose of diazepam than non-smokers)

399 a) True
  b) True
  c) True
  d) False
  e) False

It has been estimated that the incidence of alcoholism in North America and Western Europe is nearly 5 per cent of the population. Ethanol is a weak inducer of its own metabolism but is a more potent inducer of the metabolism of drugs whose principal metabolic process is via CYP450 particularly CYP2E1 and differences in rate of ethanol metabolism are principally genetic

400 a) True
   b) False   – Associated with smoking
   c) True
   d) False   – Associated with smoking
   e) False   – Associated with smoking

401 a) False   – <10 per cent
   b) True
   c) False   – Clormethiazole and benzodiazepines (long half-life) are
                   suitable sedatives
   d) True   – To avoid precipitation of acute thiamine deficiency when
                   intravenous dextrose/oral carbohydrates are administered
   e) False

402 a) False   Anabolic steroids are abused by athletes to build up muscle
   b) False   tissue
   c) True
   d) True
   e) False

403 a) True   MDMA is widely abused for its stimulant and hallucino-
   b) True   genic properties. It is metabolized by CYP2D6, which it
   c) True   inhibits for up to two weeks following a single dose. It is
   d) True   occasionally associated with hyperpyrexia, hyponatremia,
   e) True   rhabdomyolysis and coma

404 a) False   A meticulous, rapid but thorough clinical examination is
   b) True   essential not only to exclude other causes of coma or
   c) False   behaviour, but also because the symptoms and signs may
   d) True   be characteristic of certain poisons (see Table 4)
   e) False

405 a) True   – See Table 5
   b) True
   c) False
   d) False
   e) True

406 a) True   – See Table 6
   b) True
   c) True
   d) False
   e) True

407 a) False   Paracetamol and salicylate overdoses only very rarely
   b) False   cause coma acutely. Acetylcysteine is a potentially
   c) True   life-saving antidote in paracetamol overdose
   d) True
   e) False

Table 4 Clinical manifestations of some common poisons

Symptoms/signs of acute overdose	Common poisons
Coma, hypotension, flaccidity	Benzodiazepines and other hypnosedatives, alcohol
Coma, pinpoint pupils, hypoventilation	Opioids
Coma, dilated pupils, hyperreflexia, tachycardia	Tricyclic antidepressants, phenothiazines; other drugs with anticholinergic properties
Restlessness, hypertonia, hyper-reflexia, pyrexia	Amphetamines, MDMA, anticholinergic agents
Convulsions	Tricyclic antidepressants, phenothiazines, carbon monoxide, monoamine oxidase inhibitors, mefenamic acid, theophylline, hypoglycaemic agents, lithium, cyanide
Tinnitus, overbreathing, pyrexia, sweating, flushing, usually alert	Salicylates
Burns in mouth, dysphagia, abdominal pain	Corrosives, caustics, paraquat

Table 5 Common indications for emergency measurement of drug concentration

Suspected overdose	Effect on management
Paracetamol	Administration of antidotes – acetylcysteine or methionine
Iron	Administration of antidote – desferrioxamine
Methanol/ethylene glycol	Administration of antidote – ethanol or fomepizole with or without dialysis
Lithium	Dialysis
Salicylates	Simple rehydration or urinary alkalisation or dialysis
Theophylline	Necessity for ITU admission

408 **a)** False The authors recommend champagne!
b) False
c) False
d) False
e) False

Table 6 Antidotes and other specific measures

Overdose drug	Antidote/other specific measures
Paracetamol	Acetylcysteine i.v.
	Methionine p.o.
Iron	Desferrioxamine
Cyanide	Oxygen, amyl nitrate (inhalation), dicobalt edetate i.v., sodium nitrite i.v. followed by sodium thiosulphate i.v.
Benzodiazepines	Flumazenil i.v.
Beta-blockers	Atropine
	Isoprenaline
	Glucagon
Carbon monoxide	Oxygen
	Hyperbaric oxygen
Methanol/ethylene glycol	Ethanol, fomepizole
Lead (inorganic)	Sodium EDTA i.v.
	Penicillamine p.o.
	Dimercaptosuccinic acid (DMSA) i.v. or p.o.
Mercury	Dimercaptopropane sulphonate (DMPS)
	Dimercaptosuccinic acid (DMSA)
	Dimercaprol
	Penicillamine
Opioids	Naloxone
Organophosphorus insecticides	Atropine, pralidoxime
Digoxin	Digoxin-specific FAB antibody fragments
Calcium-channel blockers	Calcium chloride or gluconate i.v.
Insulin	20% dextrose i.v.
	Glucagon i.v. or i.m.

Note: DMSA, DMPS and 4-methyl-pyrazole are not licensed in the UK.

EMQ ANSWERS

409 CLINICAL MANIFESTATIONS OF DRUG OVERDOSE

1 E Coma, hypotension and flaccidity are characteristic of a significant benzodiazepine or ethanol overdose (remember to smell the breath).

2 H Coma, pinpoint pupil and hypoventilation are characteristic of opioid overdose.

3 A Coma, dilated pupils, hyperreflexia and tachycardia are characteristic of poisoning by drugs with anticholinergic properties. Tricyclic antidepressants can also cause dysrhythmias and convulsions.

4 D Other features of ecstasy (MDMA) poisoning may include: delirium, convulsions, ventricular dysrythmias, rhabdomyolysis, disseminated intravascular coagulation and adult respiratory distress syndrome.

5 G Unless comatose (rare and indicates very severe or mixed overdose) patients who have taken a salicylate overdose present feeling very unwell with tinnitus, hyperventilating, feeling hot and sweaty.

410 ANTIDOTES/OTHER SPECIFIC MEASURES IN THE MANAGEMENT OF POISONING

1 I Urinary alkalisation accelerates the urinary elimination of weak acids such as aspirin.

2 A Acetylcysteine is a potentially life-saving antidote in paracetamol poisoning. It may also be of value in carbon tetrachloride poisoning (unproven).

3 C Ethanol saturates alcohol dehydrogenase, thus blocking the conversion of methanol to the toxic formaldehyde which causes metabolic acidosis and ocular toxicity and occasionally leads to convulsions, renal failure and death. Fomepizole is a potent inhibitor of alcohol dehydrogenase. Unlike ethanol it is not sedative and has more predictable pharmacokinetics but it is not as readily available and is expensive.

4 B Desferrioxamine should be given intravenously to patients with a serum iron greater than $500 \mu g/100 \, mL$ or who have hypotension, severe lethargy, coma or convulsions.

5 J Antidotes for cyanide poisoning include nitrites (inhaled amyl nitrite and intravenous sodium nitrite), intravenous sodium thiosulphate and intravenous dicobalt edetate. Oxygen must also be administered.

CHAPTER TWELVE

PRACTICE EXAMINATION

BEST OF FIVES

1   Individuals who are slow acetylators (i.e. have a relatively low activity of hepatic *N*-acetyltransferase):

A Have a prevalence of 15–20 per cent in European caucasians
B Are more likely to develop thrombocytopenia, nephrotic syndrome and rash during gold treatment
C Are more likely to develop hepatotoxicity following halothane anaesthesia
D Are more likely to develop antinuclear antibodies during hydralazine therapy
E Are more likely to develop agranulocytosis during clozapine therapy

2   Which of the following has the shortest elimination half-life?

A Naloxone
B Morphine
C Methadone
D Fentanyl
E Remifentanil

3   Estimation of plasma/serum drug concentrations are most useful in optimizing the therapeutic dose required of:

A Warfarin
B Omeprazole
C Salbutamol
D Olanzapine
E Ciclosporin

4   Digoxin has a half-life of approximately 40 hours if renal function is normal. How long will it take to reach >90 per cent of the steady state plasma concentration?

   A 2 days
   B 7 days
   C 10 days
   D 14 days
   E 18 days

5   A 60-year-old epileptic woman who has been on the same dose of phenytoin for 20 years develops cerebellar ataxia with nystagmus. Her other medication consists of folic acid, hormone replacement therapy (HRT) and furosemide prescribed by the GP for ankle swelling and mild hypertension. She is referred to A&E. Routine investigations reveal an elevated plasma creatinine, normal plasma potassium and calcium, hypoalbuminaemia and proteinuria. The phenytoin concentration is 15 mg/L (therapeutic reference range 10–20 mg/L). A diagnosis of nephrotic syndrome is made and the cerebellar signs are attributed to phenytoin toxicity. Which of the following is likely to be correct?

   A A raised plasma creatinine interferes with the phenytoin assay, making it unreliable
   B Furosemide interferes with the blood–brain barrier, making it more permeable to phenytoin
   C Concurrent oestrogen (in the HRT) increases the CNS toxicity of phenytoin
   D The unbound phenytoin (free phenytoin) fraction is 20 per cent rather than 10 per cent
   E The cerebellar signs are more likely to be related to a cerebrovascular event

6   Which of the following drugs need *not* be avoided or only used at a reduced dose in renal failure?

   A Prednisolone
   B Netilmicin (an aminoglycoside)
   C Metformin
   D Methotrexate
   E Tinzaparin (a low molecular weight heparin, LMWH)

7   Which of the following drugs is more likely to cause hyperkalaemia than hypokalaemia in a patient with diabetes and estimated glomerular filtration rate (eGFR) within the 'normal' reference range?

   A Amphotericin
   B Prednisolone
   C LMWH
   D Salmeterol
   E Insulin

8 It is rational and advised therapeutic practice to commence treatment with the following drug using a loading dose if a rapid onset of action is required:

A Clozapine
B Zolmitriptan
C Amiodarone
D Levodopa
E Doxazosin

9 Which of the following drugs is contraindicated if there is a history of acute porphyria?

A Quinine
B Atenolol
C Oral contraceptive
D Heparin
E Amoxicillin

10 A 20-year-old man is diagnosed to have acute schizophrenia. Which of the following is an appropriate first-line treatment?

A Intravenous (i.v.) haloperidol
B Intramuscular flupentixol
C Oral olanzapine
D Oral procyclidine
E Oral fluoxetine

11 Which of the following agents if taken in overdose by a depressed patient is most likely to result in a fatal outcome?

A Amitriptyline
B Fluoxetine
C Fluvoxamine
D Paroxetine
E Citalopram

12 Which of the following drugs is likely to increase the plasma lithium concentration if co-prescribed to a patient on chronic lithium therapy?

A St John's wort
B Ibuprofen
C Phenytoin
D Haloperidol
E Sertraline

13 Which of the following is least likely to have an adverse drug interaction with phenelzine (a monoamine oxidase (MAO) inhibitor)?

A Levodopa
B Ropinirole
C Tolcapone
D Propofol
E Pseudoephedrine

14 Which of the following antiepileptic drugs is associated with visual field defects?

A Valproate
B Carbamazepine
C Lamotrigine
D Vigabatrin
E Tiagabine

15 Which of the following is the most effective in the management of absence seizures?

A Carbamazepine
B Topiramate
C Clobazam
D Phenytoin
E Ethosuximide

16 Which drug in the following list has an analgesic effect which is *not* mediated wholly or partly by binding to opioid receptors?

A Codeine
B Tramadol
C Dextropropoxyphene
D Nefopam
E Buprenorphine

17 Carbidopa when combined with levodopa:

A Inhibits the intracerebral metabolism of levodopa
B Reduces nausea and postural hypotension by permitting a lower dose of levodopa
C Cannot be prescribed with concomitant warfarin
D Delays the onset of improvement in bradykinesia
E Abolishes the 'on–off' phenomenon

18   Which of the following drugs blocks reuptake of 5-hydroxytryptamine (serotonin)?

   A Buspirone
   B Pizotifen
   C Granisetron
   D Paroxetine
   E Sumatriptan

19   Which of the following is most suitable for migraine prophylaxis in an otherwise healthy 30-year-old woman?

   A Ergotamine
   B Paracetamol
   C Propranolol
   D Carbamazepine
   E Sumatriptan

20   The following is suitable for treatment of acute dystonia as a result of metoclopramide treatment:

   A Procyclidine intravenously
   B Benzhexol orally
   C Levodopa subcutaneously
   D Bromocriptine sublingually
   E Risperidone intramuscularly

21   A 65-year-old man undergoes an orthopaedic procedure. He spends an hour in the recovery room before being returned to the ward. You are called to see him and on examination note that he is drowsy, has shallow breathing, a slow pulse and pinpoint pupils. The notes show an uneventful anaesthetic using an inhalational agent, muscle relaxant and fentanyl. In the recovery room he was breathing normally and was awake, but because of pain was initially given intravenous morphine and then intramuscular morphine before being returned to the ward. Your course of action is:

   A Call the resuscitation team
   B Give i.v. atropine
   C Give i.v. neostigmine
   D Give i.v. flumazenil
   E Give i.v. naloxone

22   A 38-year-old man with hypertension experiences a first ever attack of
     acute pain, redness and tenderness in the left first metatarsophalangeal
     joint ('podagra'). His medication is furosemide, calcium carbonate and
     irbesartan. Serum uric acid is 0.78 mmol/L (upper limit of normal for
     men 0.48 mmol/L). Which of the following is most appropriate
     pharmacotherapy?

     A Paracetamol
     B Aspirin
     C Probenecid
     D Allopurinol
     E Diclofenac

23   An 80-year-old man is taking digoxin and warfarin because of
     longstanding atrial fibrillation. He has an indwelling urinary catheter
     in situ, whilst awaiting a prostatectomy. At his pre-operation assessment
     he has a ventricular rate of 120/minute. The house officer doubles his
     daily digoxin dose and the operation is delayed one week. One week
     later he returns with nausea, vomiting, diarrhoea, abdominal pain,
     confusion, delirium and visual disturbances. The most likely cause of
     his current symptoms is:

     A Viral infection
     B Hyperkalaemia
     C Excessive prolongation of prothrombin time
     D Digoxin toxicity
     E Urinary tract infection

24   Which of the following drugs is most effective in converting a patient
     with atrial fibrillation into sinus rhythm?

     A Digoxin
     B Amiodarone
     C Atenolol
     D Lidocaine
     E Diltiazem

25 A 78-year-old man is admitted with deterioration of chronic heart failure. He is house-bound and has had three similar admissions in the past nine months. There is a history of ischaemic heart disease. His medication comprises furosemide, ramipril in full dose, valsartan, spironolactone, simvastatin and aspirin. He is dyspnoeic on minimal exertion, looks unwell, pulse 100/min regular, BP 90/70 mmHg, jugular venous pressure (JVP) is at 4 cm, gallop rhythm, chest clear, pretibial oedema. ECG shows sinus rhythm, an old inferior infarct and poor anterior R wave progression. Serum urea 15 mmol/L, creatinine 90 μmol/L, Na$^+$ 140, K$^+$ 4.6. Which of the following would be most appropriate?

A Morphine
B Hydralazine and isosorbide mononitrate
C Digoxin
D Carvedilol
E Metolazone

26 A 46-year-old businessman of Caribbean origin is found to have a total serum cholesterol concentration of 6.2 mmol/L, high-density lipoprotein (HDL) of 0.7 mmol/L and triglycerides of 9.4 mmol/L. He drinks no alcohol (ethanol) during the week but admits to eight pints of lager and up to one bottle of rum at weekends. Other chemistries are notable only for a serum glutamic oxaloacetic transaminase (SGOT) level of 72 (upper limit of normal = 42 u/L) and gamma glutamyl transferase (GGT) level of 128 (upper limit of normal = 51 u/L). Which of the following is correct?

A The low HDL can be explained by his alcohol intake
B He is at risk of pancreatitis
C A fibrate is indicated in the first instance because of mixed dyslipidaemia
D Ezetimibe would increase his low-density lipoprotein (LDL)
E Eicosapentaenoic acid is indicated to lower his total cholesterol

27 An otherwise healthy 78-year-old man is found to have a blood pressure (BP) of 168/80 at a routine check, and similar pressures are confirmed on three separate occasions despite adhering to dietary advice. Investigations including an ECG and creatinine/electrolytes are normal. Which of the following is the most appropriate next step in management?

A A 2-D echo should be obtained
B Since his diastolic BP is normal he should be reassured
C Doxazosin therapy should be initiated
D Ramipril therapy should be initiated
E Amlodipine therapy should be initiated

28 A 20-year-old woman who is 15 weeks pregnant is admitted feverish and dehydrated with acute severe asthma associated with a community-acquired pneumonia. She has a history of angioedema following a cephalosporin. Which of the following is *not* appropriate therapy?

A Rehydration with intravenous crystalloid
B High inspired oxygen concentration (FiO_2 of 40 per cent)
C Nebulized salbutamol
D Intravenous hydrocortisone
E Intravenous gentamicin

29 Which drug combination is recommended for chronic hepatitis C infection?

A Pegylated interferon alfa and lamivudine
B Pegylated interferon alfa and adefovir dipivoxil
C Pegylated interferon alfa and ribavarin
D Adefovir and lamivudine
E Oseltamivir and zanamivir

30 A 60-year-old woman has ulcerative colitis resistant to aminosalicylates and topical corticosteroids. It is decided to treat her with systemic corticosteroids. Which of the following is *not* a likely complication of the treatment?

A Osteoporosis
B Weight loss
C Diabetes
D Hypertension
E Mood changes

31 Which of the following is suitable for immediate treatment of an 18-year-old woman presenting with weight loss, tachycardia and a goitre?

A Verapamil
B ^{131}Iodine
C Carbamazepine
D Atenolol
E L-Thyroxine

32 A 62-year-old woman with type 2 diabetes, hypertension, renal impairment (creatinine 146 μmol/L) and mild congestive cardiac failure has poor diabetic control (HbA$_{1c}$ = 10.5 per cent), despite treatment with maximum doses of a sulfonylurea. Her body mass index (BMI) is 26. Which of the following would be most appropriate pharmacotherapy?

A Substitute insulin for the sulfonylurea
B Add rosiglitazone
C Add bisoprolol
D Add rimonibant
E Add metformin

33 An asymptomatic 46-year-old Indian woman is found to have an elevated serum calcium (2.80 mmol/L, corrected) at a 'well-woman' screening clinic. Other chemistries are normal, in particular phosphate is 0.8 mmol/L (normal range 0.8–1.45), and parathormone (PTH) is 5.4 pmol/L (normal range <0.9–5.4). She has a sedentary occupation in a northern UK city. Which of the following would be most suitable management?

A Alfacalcidol
B Sevelamer
C Teriparatide
D Watchful waiting (monitoring serum calcium)
E Surgical exploration of the parathyroids

34 A 24-year-old beautician has a history of chronic fatigue since an attack of infectious mononucleosis when aged 20. Her fatigue has become progressively worse. Her periods are painful, heavy and irregular. Her BP is 116/62 (supine) and 92/52 (standing). Serum Na$^+$ is 132, K$^+$ 5.5, creatinine 60 μmol/L. Which of the following would be most appropriate management?

A Lifelong fludrocortisone
B Cognitive behavioural therapy
C A course of aciclovir
D A single dose of tetracosactide for diagnosis
E Estradiol

35 A 28-year-old woman is admitted with suspected urinary sepsis (temperature 40.2°C, BP 84/50, pulse 128). She had a massive haemorrhage following the birth of her only child when she was aged 24; since then she has had no periods. Her partner says that she has been progressively listless and depressed for at least two years. There is left loin tenderness and she has no pubic or axillary hair. Which of the following would be most appropriate?

A Amoxicillin (p.o.)
B Hydrocortisone (i.v.)
C Pelvic examination
D Human menopausal gonadotrophin (follicle-stimulating hormone (FSH) + luteinizing hormone (LH))
E Triiodothyronine (i.v.)

36 A 56-year-old man with progressive, chronic renal impairment is awaiting renal replacement therapy. His treatment includes calcium carbonate tablets, furosemide, irbesartan and amlodipine. He is admitted severely unwell with a BP of 40 by palpation, pulse 112. An ECG shows a broad complex tachycardia with no P waves. Serum Ca^{2+} is 2.3 mmol/L , PO_4 1.7 mmol/L, creatinine 785 μmol/L, Na^+ 142 mmol/L, K^+ 7.4 mmol/L. Which of the following would be appropriate management?

A Amiodarone (i.v.)
B Digoxin (i.v.)
C Calcium gluconate (i.v.)
D Transvenous cardiac pacing
E Colestyramine

37 Which of the following is the systemic treatment of choice for female hirsutism?

A Tamoxifen
B Ethinylestradiol
C Norethisterone
D Cyproterone
E Finasteride

38 A history of which of the following is a contraindication to short-term HRT to prevent menopausal vasomotor symptoms and menopausal vaginitis?

A Depression
B Breast cancer
C Hysterectomy
D Chronic bronchitis
E Eczema

39 Which of the following antibacterials is most suitable for treatment of a lower urinary tract infection in a 28-year-old woman who is 10 weeks pregnant?

A Amoxicillin
B Trimethoprim
C Tetracycline
D Erythromycin
E Flucloxacillin

40 A patient presents fully conscious with acute falciparum malaria following a visit to Nigeria. Which of the following treatments is most appropriate?

A Chloroquine
B Proguanil and atovaquone
C Primaquine
D Pyrimethamine
E Hydroxychloroquine

41 Which of the following drugs causes the most significant inhibition of metabolism of rifabutin?

A Zidovudine
B Ritonavir
C Enfuvirtide
D Nevirapine
E St John's wort

42 A 42-year-old woman has widely disseminated colon cancer. Her main symptom is pain from a spinal crush fracture, incompletely suppressed by oral morphine. She is also troubled by constipation, nausea and occasional vomiting. Which of the following is true?

A Fentanyl patches would not cause nausea at analgesic doses
B Cisplatin prolongs survival
C Radiotherapy to the primary with adjunctive chemotherapy is the treatment mainstay
D Biopsy of the fractured vertebra is indicated
E Intercostal nerve block should be arranged

43 Which of the following drugs used in cancer chemotherapy is most likely to be associated with cerebellar dysfunction?

A Cytosine arabinoside (cytarabine)
B Cyclophosphamide
C Mitoxantrone
D Bleomycin
E Vincristine

44 Which of the following cytotoxic drugs is least likely to cause emesis during chemotherapy?

A Cisplatin
B Dacarbazine
C Doxorubicin
D Mustine
E Vincristine

45 A 25-year-old woman suffers a bee sting and within a few minutes she notices a blotchy rash appearing on her body. She is taken to A&E where her BP is 90/60 mmHg. The most appropriate immediate therapy would be:

A Oral antihistamine (chlorphenamine 4 mg)
B Intravenous adrenaline (10 mL of 1:10 000)
C Intravenous steroid (hydrocortisone 200 mg)
D Intramuscular adrenaline (0.5 mL of 1:1000)
E Inhaled salbutamol via nebulizer

46 Which of the following is most effective as a topical agent for a candida infection of the skin?

A Griseofulvin
B Beclometasone
C Aciclovir
D Amphotericin
E Nystatin

47 Which of the following is suitable for initial treatment of acute glaucoma?

A Timolol
B Pilocarpine
C Mannitol
D Tropicamide
E Latanoprost

48 Which of the following is the antidote of first choice in the treatment of potentially fatal paracetamol overdose?

A Methionine
B Acetylcysteine
C Naloxone
D Dicobalt edetate
E Flumazenil

49 Which of the following 'overdoses' is most commonly associated with respiratory alkalosis, but when more severe a metabolic acidosis?

A Methanol
B Lead
C Paracetamol
D Salicylate
E Codeine

50 The following is most suitable for thromboembolic prophylaxis in a patient with a left ventricular aneurysm following a myocardial infarction three months ago:

A Intravenous heparin
B Subcutaneous enoxaparin
C Oral warfarin
D Oral aspirin
E Oral aspirin + clopidogrel

Answers: see pages 202–207

PROBLEM SOLVING QUESTIONS

PROBLEM 1 A PATIENT WITH TYPE 2 DIABETES WHO PRESENTS WITH CONGESTIVE CARDIAC FAILURE

Question 51

A 61-year-old woman with type 2 diabetes presents to her GP with two months progressive fatigue, effort dyspnoea and ankle swelling. She is obese and has been controlled with diet alone since diabetes was diagnosed at age 58. Her BP is 142/92 and there are signs of congestive cardiac failure. An echocardiogram confirms poor left ventricular function with a large area of anterior hypokinesia. Fasting blood glucose is 10.2 mmol/L and HbA$_{1c}$ 9.2 per cent, total cholesterol 4.8 mmol/L, HDL 0.9 mmol/L and triglyceride 1.2 mmol/L; creatinine is 92 μmol/L, serum electrolytes are normal. Management would appropriately include:

A Referral for cardiac catheterization
B Clopidogrel
C Ramipril
D Furosemide
E Rosiglitazone

Question 52

Initially she improves on treatment with metformin, simvastatin, valsartan and aspirin but two weeks later she is brought to hospital, severely ill. She is pale and shocked with a systolic BP of 76, an ECG shows Q waves in I, AVL, V1–3 and non-specific T wave changes. Urinalysis shows 1$^+$ ketones, 3$^+$ glucose, arterial blood gas (ABG) shows a pH of 6.9, oxygen saturation is 94 per cent breathing air, her temperature is 37°C, haemoglobin 12.0, white cell count 9000 with a normal differential, C reactive protein (CRP) <5, creatine kinase (CK) = 450 u/L (normal range 24–170), glucose 18.6 mmol/L. Plausible differential diagnoses include:

A Acute gastrointestinal blood loss
B Diabetic ketoacidosis
C Lactic acidosis
D Non-ST elevation myocardial infarction (NSTEMI)
E Acute rhabdomyolysis

Question 53

Management on the ITU would appropriately include:

A Discontinuation of metformin
B Intravenous infusion of adrenaline
C Hyperbaric O$_2$
D Intravenous insulin
E Intravenous pantoprazole

PROBLEM 2 CARPAL TUNNEL SYNDROME

Question 54

A 43-year-old vegetarian woman presents with symptoms of carpal tunnel syndrome (right worse than left). There is a family history of type 1 diabetes. Her heart rate is 52 and she has several large patches of vitiligo. Investigations include total serum cholesterol 7.2 mmol/L, HDL 1.2 mmol/L, triglycerides 0.8 mmol/L, CK 150 u/L (normal range 24–170), haemoglobin 11.6 with macrocytic red cells present on the film. Immediate management should include:

A Vitamin B12 injection
B Surgical referral for right wrist decompression
C Triiodothyronine
D Simvastatin
E Measurement of serum thyrotropin (TSH)

Question 55

Serum vitamin B12 comes back as 160 ng/L (normal range 150–750) and intrinsic factor antibodies are positive. She improves initially with appropriate therapy but one month later develops symptoms of classical angina. Her heart rate is 72 and regular and the examination otherwise unremarkable. An ECG is normal. Management should include:

A Bone marrow examination
B Atenolol
C Measurement of serum thyrotropin
D Simvastatin
E Cardiological referral

Question 56

Walking home from the consultation with her GP she becomes acutely unwell with chest pain and palpitations. She is taken by ambulance to the emergency department. Her BP is 126/68. An ECG shows heart rate of 96 and is otherwise normal except for some non-specific T wave changes. Immediate management should include:

A Ciclosporin
B Thrombolysis
C Aspirin (300 mg p.o.)
D Carbimazole
E Beta blockade

PROBLEM 3 LOSS OF BLOOD PRESSURE CONTROL

Question 57

A 67-year-old man was diagnosed with essential hypertension aged 52 at which time investigations were normal. He was treated with amlodipine and atenolol with good control until the most recent three readings of around 160/100 over the past three months. He is otherwise well in himself but is awaiting orthopaedic assessment because of osteoarthrosis in his left hip. His only other regular medication is naproxen for hip pain. He has 2^+ ankle oedema but no other signs of congestive heart failure. Serum creatinine is 320 μmol/L. Serum cholesterol is 4.6 mmol/L, urine protein 2^+. Immediate management should include:

A Substitution of atenolol with an angiotensin-converting enzyme (ACE) inhibitor
B Discontinuation of amlodipine
C Substitution of regular paracetamol for naproxen
D Renal ultrasound
E Measurement of random renin and aldosterone

Question 58

Following appropriate changes to his medication, his BP improves to around 150/95 and his serum creatinine falls to 280 μmol/L. Pain in his hip becomes more troublesome. A magnetic resonance angiogram of the renal arteries shows irregularities of both renal arteries. Irbesartan is commenced.

A This may protect residual renal function
B This may precipitate acute renal failure
C A statin is indicated
D Low-dose aspirin is contraindicated
E Codeine could usefully be prescribed

Question 59

His BP improves to around 130/80 as does the pain in his hip, but he becomes constipated and his ankle swelling persists.

A Watchful waiting and dietary advice are appropriate
B Hip replacement is contraindicated
C Angioplasty of renal arteries is indicated
D Substitution of modified release verapamil for amlodipine is indicated to improve ankle swelling
E Senna may be useful

PROBLEM 4 DEEP VEIN THROMBOSIS IN PREGNANCY

Question 60

A 28-year-old woman develops a deep vein thrombosis in week 34 of her first pregnancy.

A LMWH is contraindicated because it crosses the placenta
B Warfarin should be started only after delivery
C Breastfeeding will be contraindicated
D Vaginal delivery is contraindicated
E Antiplatelet therapy with aspirin is indicated

Question 61

Two days following delivery she becomes acutely short of breath. BP is 104/64, respiratory rate 24; pulse 128 irregular, there is a gallop rhythm, oxygen saturation is 88 per cent, an ECG confirms atrial fibrillation.

A Computerized tomography (CT) pulmonary angiogram is appropriate
B Post-partum cardiomyopathy is the probable underlying diagnosis
C Digoxin is appropriate
D Serum thyrotropin should be measured
E DC cardioversion is indicated

Question 62

Following discharge:

A Warfarin is indicated
B Oral contraception is contraindicated in the long term
C Electrophysiological mapping of pre-excitation pathways should be undertaken
D Anticoagulation should be life-long
E Residual effort dyspnoea could be due to pulmonary hypertension

PROBLEM 5 CHILD WITH HEADACHE, VOMITING, FEVER AND NECK STIFFNESS

Question 63

A 4-year-old child presents to A&E complaining of a 6-hour history of gradually increasing and severe headache and vomiting. On examination, she has a temperature of 38.5°C, and marked neck stiffness, but no rash is present. Fundoscopy proves impossible due to severe photophobia. Initial management should include:

A Immediate lumbar puncture
B Oral co-amoxiclav
C CT head scan
D Intravenous ceftriaxone
E Antibiotics should not be started until a lumbar puncture has been performed and cerebrospinal fluid sent for bacteriological analysis

Question 64

A CT head scan reveals no evidence of raised pressure, and is otherwise unremarkable. A subsequent lumbar puncture reveals a purulent meningitis, with high neutrophil count, raised protein and depressed glucose levels. Microscopy reveals the presence of *Haemophilus influenzae*, and this is confirmed on subsequent culture to be *H. influenzae* type b. Further management should include:

A Ceftriaxone for 5 days
B Ceftriaxone for 10 days
C Amoxicillin for 10 days
D Metronidazole
E Rifampicin

Question 65

She makes a good recovery. However, soon after the antibiotic is stopped, she develops watery diarrhoea associated with abdominal pain. Two days later, she has fever and bloody diarrhoea (frequency 20 times per day). Appropriate management should now include:

A Restarting the original antibiotic
B Intravenous vancomycin
C Oral metronidazole
D Intravenous fluid replacement
E Corticosteroid therapy

Answers: see pages 208–210

ANSWERS

ANSWERS TO 'BEST OF FIVES'

1   **D**   Rapid acetylator status has a prevalence of 45–50 per cent in European caucasians. Individuals who are 'rapid acetylators' are more likely to develop peripheral neuropathy during isoniazid therapy.

2   **E**   Remifentanil has an elimination half-life of 5–7 minutes, naloxone 30–80 minutes, morphine 90–120 minutes, fentanyl 2–4 hours, methadone 15–55 hours. If naloxone is used to reverse opioid agonist effects, repeat dose/doses/infusion may be necessary to outlast the opioid effect, with the exception of remifentanil (and possibly alfentanil which has a half-life of 40–140 minutes).

3   **E**   Ciclosporin is a potent immunosuppressant which is of particular value in organ transplantation. It has little effect on the bone marrow, but is nephrotoxic. There is considerable interindividual variability in its pharmacokinetics.

4   **B**   If a constant dose of a drug is administered at intervals less than its half-life, the average concentration will rise to a plateau (see *Textbook of Clinical Pharmacology and Therapeutics*, Chapter 3, Figure 3.3). After one half-life (in the case of digoxin 40 hours), the plasma concentration will be 50 per cent of the plateau (steady state concentration) after two half-lives 75 per cent, three half-lives 87.5 per cent and after four half-lives 93.75 per cent; 4×40 hours = 6.6 days.

5   **D**   Hypoalbuminaemia will result in an increased ratio of unbound:bound (i.e. active:inactive) phenytoin in plasma. Therapeutic drug monitoring assays routinely measure total plasma drug and do not differentiate between bound and unbound drug. Hence in conditions where hypoalbuminaemia exists (e.g. nephrotic syndrome and pregnancy) the usual therapeutic concentration range is inappropriate. In severe renal failure endogenous substances that accumulate due to renal failure may also displace drugs from protein-binding sites.

6   **A**   Prednisolone metabolic clearance is not significantly altered in renal dysfunction. Netilmicin, an aminoglycoside, and methotrexate are nephrotoxic and accumulate in renal failure. Tinzaparin, unlike heparin, depends on renal elimination. Metformin is associated with a greatly increased risk of lactic acidosis in renal impairment.

7   **C**   Inhibition of aldosterone secretion by heparin, including LMWHs, can cause hyperkalaemia. Those with diabetes, chronic renal failure,

acidosis and those on potassium-sparing drugs are most at risk. The other drugs listed are associated with hypokalaemia.

8   C   It takes approximately four times the half-life to reach 93.75 per cent of steady state plasma concentration. A loading dose is rational for a drug with a long half-life if a rapid onset of action is required, the effect is related to plasma concentration and administering the loading dose is safe.

9   C   Acute illness is precipitated by drugs because of inherited enzyme deficiencies in the pathway of haem synthesis. Drug-induced exacerbations of acute porphyria (neurological, psychiatric, cardiovascular and gastrointestinal disturbances that are occasionally fatal) are accompanied by increased urinary excretion of 5-aminolevulinic acid (ALA) and porphobilinogen.

10   C   An oral atypical antipsychotic drug (e.g. amisulpride, olanzapine, quetiapine, risperidone, zotepine) is considered by the National Institute for Health and Clinical Excellence (NICE) the treatment option of choice for managing an acute schizophrenic episode when discussion with the individual is not possible. Atypical antipsychotics have the advantage that extrapyramidal adverse effects (associated with increased binding to and receptor occupancy of D_2 receptors) are much less common than with the conventional D_2 antagonists.

11   A   Amitriptyline is an effective, sedative, tricyclic antidepressant. It is much more dangerous in overdose (coma, convulsions and dysrhythmias) than the selective serotonin reuptake inhibitors (SSRIs) listed here.

12   B   Concomitant non-steroidal anti-inflammatory drugs (NSAIDs) such as ibuprofen, ACE inhibitors, angiotensin receptor blockers (ARBs) and diuretics cause increased lithium concentrations.

13   D   Diet and drug interactions are a danger with MAO inhibitors. The tyramine reaction is much less of a danger with moclobemide (reversible, selective MAO type A) inhibitor and selegeline (selective MAO type B inhibitor).

14   D   Vigabatrin, a structural analogue of gamma-aminobutyric acid (GABA), inhibits GABA transaminase, increasing cerebral GABA (an inhibitory neurotransmitter). It is associated with visual field defects in approximately one-third of patients in whom it is used. These defects may persist in spite of drug withdrawal.

15   E   Ethosuxamide and valproate are regarded as the first-line drugs for absence seizures.

16   D   Nefopam is chemically and pharmacologically unrelated to other analgesics. It inhibits 5HT uptake and potentiates adrenergic pathways that operate the gate mechanism for pain.

17 **B** Carbidopa, a peripheral dopa decarboxylase inhibitor, inhibits the extracerebral metabolism of levodopa to dopamine.

18 **D** Paroxetine is an SSRI. Indications include major depression, obsessive–compulsive disorder, panic disorder, post-traumatic stress disorder and anxiety. Extrapyramidal reactions (including orofacial dystonias) have been reported with paroxetine.

19 **C** Lipid-soluble beta blockers such as propranolol, which penetrate the blood–brain barrier, are useful for prophylaxis. Ergotamine and sumatriptan are used for treatment of an acute migraine attack (ergotamine has now largely been superseded by drugs such as the triptans), and are not useful for regular use to prevent migraine attacks.

20 **A** Antimuscarinic drugs are useful for reducing the symptoms of parkinsonism induced by dopamine antagonist drugs such as the antipsychotics, and given parenterally are the drugs of choice for acute dystonic reactions caused by dopamine antagonists. Parenteral benzodiazepines are also effective in acute drug-induced dystonia. Levodopa and bromocriptine are only available as oral preparations.

21 **E** Intravenous naloxone should immediately reverse the signs of opioid overdose.

22 **E** Diclofenac is effective for the acute inflammation of gout. Paracetamol is less anti-inflammatory and ordinary doses of aspirin can increase plasma uric acid. Probenecid (uricosuric) and allopurinol (blocks uric acid synthesis) are contraindicated during the acute attack.

23 **D** The symptoms described are characteristic of digoxin toxicity.

24 **B** Amiodarone has class III antidysrhythmic activity, and can be used for chemical cardioversion of atrial fibrillation. Digoxin has some effect in slowing resting heart rate in patients with atrial fibrillation, but does not convert patients to sinus rhythm. Beta blockers are good for rate control in atrial fibrillation, but (with the exception of sotalol) do not convert patients to sinus rhythm. Lidocaine is only effective for ventricular tachydysrhythmias. Diltiazem, like verapamil, is of some use in rate control and in prevention of paroxysms of atrial fibrillation.

25 **C** He is unstable and hypotensive so beta blockade is not appropriate. Although unstable he does not have signs of pulmonary oedema and morphine is not indicated. The raised urea with normal creatinine suggests pre-renal impairment which would be worsened by metolazone. Digoxin improves symptoms and reduces readmission rates in patients with severe heart failure.

26 B He is drinking excessively and has marked hypertriglyceridaemia. Alcohol increases HDL. He would be at risk of rhabdomyolysis on a fibrate and the first line should be to stop drinking alcohol. Ezetimibe has little effect on HDL and eicosapentaenoic acid has little or no effect on total cholesterol or LDL.

27 E Isolated systolic hypertension is common in the elderly, in whom it is an important cardiovascular risk factor. Lowering systolic pressure reduces this excess risk. Renin is seldom elevated in this age group and a calcium antagonist or diuretic is appropriate initial drug treatment.

28 E The appropriate antibacterial in this situation is a macrolide, e.g. clarithromycin or erythromycin.

29 C In hepatitis C the liver function may remain normal for months to years. The course of the liver damage often fluctuates. Up to 60 per cent of patients with hepatitis C do not clear the virus spontaneously. Chronic liver disease, cirrhosis and hepatocellular carcinoma may develop. NICE has recommended peginterferon alfa and ribavarin for chronic hepatitis C with caveats.

30 B Chronic systemic corticosteroid therapy causes iatrogenic Cushing's syndrome. Weight gain is characteristic.

31 D She probably has Graves' disease. A beta blocker will improve her symptoms while the results of thyroid function tests are awaited. If confirmed, prolonged specific antithyroid treatment with carbimazole (or a related drug) will be indicated. ^{131}Iodine-treatment may be useful if this fails provided pregnancy is excluded/avoided.

32 A Approximately one-third of people with type 2 diabetes benefit from insulin. Glitazones are contraindicated in heart failure, beta blockers are likely to worsen her diabetic control, she is not obese and metformin is contraindicated in renal impairment and congestive heart failure.

33 D The probable diagnosis is mild primary hyperparathyroidism since PTH is inappropriately high for the plasma calcium concentration, and phosphate is at the lower end of the normal range. Alfacalcidol or teriparatide would further increase plasma calcium and sevelamer (phosphate binder) is also contraindicated. Surgery would only be appropriate if Ca^{2+} was to rise further and symptoms occur.

34 D The probable diagnosis is Addison's disease. This may be confirmed by a stimulation test with tetracosactide. Definitive treatment would be with glucocorticosteroid replacement supplemented by fludrocortisone (mineralocorticoid) only if necessary. Her gynaecological symptoms should be reassessed when Addison's disease has been dealt with.

35 **B** The history suggests Sheehan's syndrome with superimposed acute pyelonephritis. In addition to i.v. antibiotics she should be treated urgently with i.v. hydrocortisone since she may well be hypoadrenal (from lack of pituitary ACTH) in addition to hypogonadal (from lack of FSH/LH) and possibly hypothyroid (from lack of TSH). Unlike glucocorticosteroid replacement, replacement of sex hormones and thyroid hormone is less urgent and should await investigation.

36 **C** Calcium gluconate (i.v.) is effective in urgent treatment of broad complex tachycardia caused by hyperkalaemia. A cation-exchange resin such as calcium resonium (rather than a bile acid-binding resin such as colestyramine) might subsequently be used while arranging urgent dialysis.

37 **D** Cyproterone is an anti-androgen. In women it has been used to treat hyperandrogenic effects (often seen in polycystic ovary disease) including acne, hirsutism and male pattern baldness.

38 **B** If HRT is contraindicated as in breast cancer, clonidine may be used to reduce vasomotor symptoms.

39 **A** Amoxicillin is suitable for treatment for lower urinary tract infections, pending results of urine cultures, and is not harmful to the embryo or fetus. Tetracycline, erythromycin and flucloxacillin are not good choices for urine infections, and tetracycline can affect skeletal development (this has been seen in animal studies) and causes dental discolouration in the fetus. Trimethoprim is potentially teratogenic in the first trimester, because of its action at inhibiting folate biosynthesis (dihydrofolate reductase).

40 **B** Most falciparum malaria is chloroquine resistant these days. Quinine is a suitable treatment, and should be given for 5–7 days followed by a 7-day course of doxycycline or a single dose of Fansidar® (pyrimethamine with sulfadoxine). Malarone® (proguanil combined with atovaquone) is a good alternative treatment, its advantages being that it need only be given for 3 days and does not need to be followed by any other drugs.

41 **B** Rifabutin is a rifamycin which is active against mycobacteria. In patients with low CD4 count it is indicated as prophylaxis against *Mycobacterium avium* complex infections. Ritonavir, an anti-HIV protease inhibitor, inhibits drug metabolism of CYP3A substrates and some CYP2D6 substrates. It increases the risk of uveitis if prescribed with rifabutin. The combination should be avoided.

42 **E** Intercostal nerve block would promptly alleviate her main symptom. Fentanyl patches could be better than oral morphine because she is vomiting. Colon cancer is not very sensitive to radiotherapy or

chemotherapy although radiotherapy to the presumed vertebral
metastasis could be useful symptomatically in the medium term.

43 A Cytarabine interferes with pyrimidine synthesis and is used in the
induction of remission in acute myeloblastic leukaemia. Its main toxicity is myelosuppresion. With high doses approximately 10 per cent
of patients have cerebellar toxicity.

44 E Vincristine, and other vinca alkaloids, are only weakly emetogenic.
Peripheral and autonomic neuropathies are associated with vincristine. All vinca alkaloids are very irritant and can cause severe
local tissue damage if extravasation occurs.

45 D Intramuscular adrenaline 500 µg (0.5 mL adrenaline injection 1 in
1000) may be life-saving in acute anaphylaxis. The dose is repeated if
necessary at 5-minute intervals.

46 E Nystatin, ketoconazole, clotrimazole, miconazole, terbinafine and
amorolfine may all be used topically for candida infections of the
skin, vulvovaginitis or balanitis. Systemic therapy may be required
in refractory cases. Consider underlying diabetes mellitus.

47 C Acute glaucoma is a medical emergency, and initial treatment
should be with i.v. mannitol, usually with the addition of a carbonic
anhydrase inhibitor (i.v. acetazolamide or topical dorzolamide). This
can then supplemented with either a topical beta blocker (e.g. timolol) or a topical cholinergic agonist (e.g. pilocarpine), or both.
Latanoprost is a prostaglandin $F_{2\alpha}$ analogue, which can be used topically in the more chronic situation, in patients who are intolerant of
beta blockers or as add-on therapy when the initial response has
been inadequate. Tropicamide is a muscarinic antagonist used to
dilate the pupil for fundoscopic examination, and raises intraocular
pressure, so is contraindicated in this situation.

48 B Intravenous acetylcysteine is potentially life-saving following paracetamol overdose.

49 D In salicylate overdose blood gases and arterial pH normally reveal a
mixed metabolic acidosis and respiratory alkalosis. Respiratory alkalosis is due to direct stimulation of the respiratory centre. Metabolic
acidosis is due to uncoupling of oxidative phosphorylation and lactic acidosis. If acidosis predominates, the prognosis is poor.

50 C Patients with a left ventricular aneurysm are at high risk of forming
intra-aneurysmal clot and subsequent arterial embolic disease, and
in the absence of compelling contraindications should be anticoagu-
lated with warfarin. Antiplatelet treatment is of little or no use in
this situation.

ANSWERS TO PROBLEM SOLVING QUESTIONS

PROBLEM 1

Question 51, Answers: T F T T F

Question 52, Answers: T F T T F

Question 53, Answers: T T F T T

Comment

Initial treatment with metformin is problematic in view of congestive heart failure (CHF). Her acute deterioration could have been precipitated by a gastrointestinal bleed (aspirin) or acute ischaemia and appears to be complicated by acidosis – probably lactic acidosis (predisposed by metformin) in view of only 1^+ urine ketones and only moderately elevated blood glucose. This is not the presentation of rhabdomyolysis and CK is only moderately elevated. Hyperbaric O_2 is not evidence based and not available in ITU.

PROBLEM 2

Question 54, Answers: F F F F T

Question 55, Answers: F T T T T

Question 56, Answers: F F T F T

Comment

Carpal tunnel syndrome is a common presentation of hypothyroidism (confirmed by measuring serum thyrotropin). This can cause a raised serum cholesterol, macrocytosis and mildly raised CK. There is a family history of autoimmune disease and she may well be developing vitamin B12 deficiency in addition to hypothyroidism. Appropriate medical treatment is oral thyroxine. This may obviate the need for surgery and may correct her dyslipidaemia. Thyroxine has a long half-life so occurrence of angina after four weeks treatment when accumulation will have occurred and serum levels have increased, suggests that she may have underlying ischaemic heart disease which has been masked by bradycardia and hypothyroidism. The dose of thyroxine should be reduced and a beta blocker added. The acute event is strongly suggestive of an acute coronary syndrome. Aspirin 300 mg rapidly blocks platelet cyclo-oxygenase (COX) and is the appropriate starting dose in this acute setting. Carbimazole blocks thyroid hormone synthesis so would not antagonize exogenous thyroxine.

PROBLEM 3

Question 57, Answers: F F T T F

Question 58, Answers: T T T F T

Question 59, Answers: T F F F T

Comment

Possible explanations of loss of BP control and occurrence of renal impairment include onset of renal disease (e.g. renal artery stenosis or obstructive uropathy) and/or inhibition of renal COX by naproxen. Paracetamol, codeine and low-dose aspirin do not share these effects on BP and renal function. Atenolol suppresses renin, making measurement of this uninformative. An ACE inhibitor or ARB can protect against progressive renal dysfunction, but can precipitate acute renal failure if there is haemodynamically significant bilateral renal artery stenosis (possible in view of the irregularities seen). Angioplasty is not indicated unless renal function deteriorates and is not particularly effective in atheromatous disease. Verapamil is less likely to cause oedema than amlodipine but will make constipation worse and may precipitate heart failure with concomitant atenolol.

PROBLEM 4

Question 60, Answers: F T F F F

Question 61, Answers: T F T T F

Question 62, Answers: T T F F T

Comment

LMWH does not cross the placenta. Warfarin is contraindicated in the last trimester because of the risk of intracranial haemorrhage in the infant and of maternal bleeding. After delivery warfarin can be used and appears safe in breastfeeding. Antiplatelet therapy is inadequate prophylaxis in deep vein thrombosis (DVT). The acute episode following delivery is presumably due to pulmonary embolism which may have precipitated atrial fibrillation but other causes of atrial fibrillation remain possible. Serum thyroxine is difficult to interpret peripartum but serum thyrotropin can be interpreted (a depressed level would signal probable hyperthyroidism). Anticoagulation would not need to be indefinite since DVT occurred in the setting of pregnancy. If there has been a large pulmonary embolus, this may cause pulmonary hypertension.

PROBLEM 5

Question 63, Answers: F F T T F

Comment

If bacterial meningitis is suspected, as in this case, i.v. antibiotic should be started without waiting for microscopy/culture results from the cerebrospinal fluid, due to the often rapid progression of the disease with potentially devastating consequences. Intravenous ceftriaxone is a good initial broad-spectrum treatment, pending bacteriology results. Since fundoscopy was not possible, a lumbar puncture should not be performed until a CT scan has confirmed the absence of raised intracranial pressure, due to the possibility of coning being induced in this situation.

Question 64, Answers: F T F F T

Comment

H. influenzae meningitis should be treated with a third-generation cephalosporin intravenously for at least 10 days. Chloramphenicol can be substituted where there is a history of anaphylaxis to penicillin or to cephalosporins, or if the organism is resistant to cephalosporins. For *H. influenzae* type b, rifampicin should be given for 4 days before hospital discharge, to prevent carriage. Metronidazole is active against anaerobic organisms.

Question 65, Answers: F F T T F

Comment

This patient has developed pseudomembranous colitis, due to *Clostridium difficile* overgrowth in the gut, whose toxin gives rise to this condition. It can occur following treatment with any antibiotic, but appears to be a particular hazard with clindamycin and cephalosporins. Oral metronidazole or oral vancomycin are used as specific treatment.